Michelle J. Lawson

The Anti-Skin Cancer Cookbook

For both men and women over 40

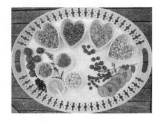

Delicious Recipes and Strategies for Preventing and Treating Skin-Cancer

(Melanoma)

Copyright & Disclaimer

Dedication

To my loving husband,

This book is dedicated to you with all my heart. Your unwavering support, encouragement, and belief in me have been the driving force behind the completion of this book. You have been my rock, my confidant, and my inspiration throughout this journey.

Your patience, understanding, and sacrifices have made it possible for me to pursue my dreams and reach this significant milestone in my life. Your love and support have given me the strength and courage to overcome every obstacle and challenge that came my way.

With all my love and appreciation,

Michelle.

Table of Contents

Introduction

Understanding Skin Cancer (Melanoma)and Its Causes

Skin cancer is one of the most widely recognized sorts of cancer, with melanoma being the most forceful type of skin cancer. Melanoma emerges from the color-delivering cells (melanocytes) in the skin and can foster any place on the body, including regions not presented to the sun. Understanding the causes, risk variables, and prevention strategies for melanoma is significant for early detection and effective treatment.

Causes of Melanoma

The specific cause of melanoma is unknown, yet a few variables are known to expand the risk of fostering this cancer. The main risk factor is openness to bright (UV) radiation from the sun or fake sources, like tanning beds.

At the point when skin is presented to UV radiation, it harms the DNA in skin cells and can prompt changes that cause cells to develop and separate wildly, shaping cancerous growths.

Different variables that might expand the risk of melanoma incorporate a family background of the infection, having numerous moles or abnormal moles, having a light complexion, red or light hair, and light-hued eyes. Individuals with a debilitated safe framework, for example, the people who have gotten an organ relocation or are taking meds that smother the insusceptible framework, are likewise at a higher risk of creating melanoma.

Signs and Symptoms of Melanoma

Melanoma often creates another mole or a current mole that adjusts in size, shape, or variety. The ABCDE rule can assist with recognizing potential signs of melanoma:

A - Imbalance: One portion of the mole doesn't match the other half.

B - Border irregularity: The edges of the mole are worn out, indented, or obscured.

C - Variety: The mole has lopsided shading, with shades of dark, brown, and tan, or even white, red, or blue.

D - Diameter: The mole is bigger than the size of a pencil eraser.

E - Evolving: The mole is changing in size, shape, variety, or level.

Different signs and symptoms of melanoma incorporate an irritation that doesn't mend, a mole that becomes excruciating or bothersome, or a dull streak under a fingernail or toenail.

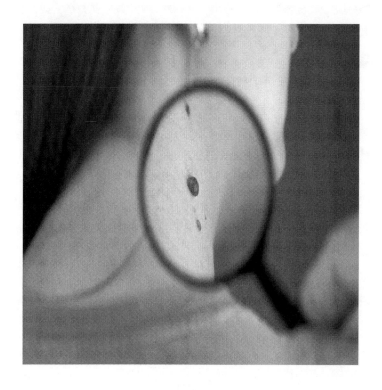

<u>Prevention and Early Detection of Melanoma</u>

Prevention and early detection are fundamental for lessening the risk of melanoma and working on the possibilities of effective treatment. The American Cancer Society prescribes the accompanying strategies to forestall melanoma:

Safeguard your skin from the sun: Keep away from sun openness during top hours (10 a.m. to 4 p.m.) and wear defensive attire, like long-sleeved shirts, caps, and shades. Utilize a wide range of sunscreen with an SPF of something like 30, and apply it liberally to all uncovered skin, including your lips and the highest points of your ears. Reapply sunscreen at regular intervals or all the more much of the time assuming you are swimming or perspiring.

Abstain from tanning beds: Tanning beds produce UV radiation that can cause skin harm and increment the risk of melanoma.

Look at your skin consistently: Take a look at your skin for new moles or changes in existing moles one time per month.

Utilize a mirror to check hard-to-see regions, like your scalp, back, and rear end. If you notice any changes, see a dermatologist for a skin test.

Know your risk: Converse with your medical care supplier about your risk of melanoma and whether you ought to have standard skin tests.

- Stay away from openness to counterfeit wellsprings of UV radiation: This incorporates tanning lights and stalls.

<u>Treatment of Melanoma</u>

The treatment of melanoma includes a multidisciplinary approach that incorporates a medical procedure, chemotherapy, radiation treatment, and immunotherapy.

The medical procedure is the essential treatment for melanoma. The objective of medical procedures is to eliminate the cancerous tissue and an edge of solid tissue encompassing it to forestall a repeat. The kind of medical procedure relies upon the size, area, and phase of the melanoma.

For little melanomas, an excisional biopsy is often performed, which includes eliminating the whole growth and an edge of ordinary skin. For bigger melanomas, wide extraction medical procedures might be fundamental, which includes eliminating cancer and a more extensive room for error of skin and basic tissue. At times, lymph hubs in the space of the melanoma may likewise be eliminated to decide whether cancer has spread.

If the melanoma has spread to different parts of the body, chemotherapy might be suggested. Chemotherapy includes the utilization of medications to kill cancer cells. It may very well be given orally or intravenously. Chemotherapy is often utilized in a blend with different treatments, like a medical procedure or radiation treatment. The decision of chemotherapy relies upon the phase of the melanoma, the area of cancer, and the patient's general well-being.

Radiation treatment is one more treatment choice for melanoma. It includes the utilization of high-energy X-beams to kill cancer cells. Radiation treatment is often utilized after a medical procedure to obliterate any leftover cancer cells. It might likewise be utilized as a palliative treatment to ease symptoms caused by melanoma that has spread to different pieces of the body, like bone torment or migraines.

Immunotherapy is a fresher treatment for melanoma that has shown promising outcomes. It includes the utilization of medications that assist the body's invulnerable framework with battling cancer. The most widely recognized sort of immunotherapy for melanoma is designated spot inhibitors, which block proteins that cancer cells use to avoid the resistant framework. Immunotherapy is often utilized in cutting-edge melanoma that has spread to different pieces of the body.

It might likewise be utilized as an adjuvant treatment to lessen the risk of repeating after a medical procedure.

Notwithstanding these treatments, there are a few different treatments that might be utilized to treat melanoma. These incorporate designated treatment, which includes the utilization of medications that target explicit proteins in cancer cells; intralesional treatment, which includes infusing drugs straightforwardly into the growth; and cryotherapy, which includes freezing the cancer cells with fluid nitrogen.

The decision of treatment for melanoma relies upon a few variables, including the phase of the cancer, the area of the melanoma, and the patient's general well-being. The earlier the melanoma is recognized, the better the possibilities of effective treatment. Thus, it is essential to perform normal skin self-tests and have any dubious moles or injuries assessed by a medical services professional.

The Link Between Diet and Skin Cancer

As we all know, skin cancer is a serious worry in this day and age. As per the American Cancer Society, skin cancer is the most well-known type of cancer in the US, with over 5 million new cases analyzed every year. While various elements can add to the improvement of skin cancer, one of the most significant is diet.

There is a developing collection of examinations that proposes that specific dietary examples and supplements can either increment or decline a singular's risk of creating skin cancer. In this segment of the cookbook, we will investigate the connection between diet and skin cancer and furnish you with certain tips on the best way to change your diet to lessen your risk of fostering this possibly destructive sickness.

Above all, it's essential to comprehend that there are two primary kinds of skin cancer: melanoma and non-melanoma. Melanoma is a more serious type of skin cancer that can spread to other pieces of the body whenever left untreated. Non-melanoma skin cancers, like basal cell carcinoma and squamous cell carcinoma, are for the most part less forceful however can in any case be hazardous if not gotten early.

So how precisely does diet influence the improvement of these kinds of skin cancer? One of the key ways is through the admission of specific supplements, like antioxidants and omega-3 unsaturated fats. Antioxidants are intensely tracked down in many leafy foods that assist to shield the body from the harmful impacts of free extremists, which can add to the improvement of cancer. Omega-3 unsaturated fats are a kind of solid fat that can be tracked down in greasy fish, nuts, and seeds. They have been displayed to have mitigating properties, which can likewise assist with decreasing the risk of cancer.

Another significant component to consider is the admission of specific sorts of food varieties. For instance, a diet that is high in handled and refined food varieties, for example, sweet tidbits and cheap food, has been connected to an expanded risk of skin cancer. Then again, a diet that is wealthy in entire food sources, like natural products, vegetables, entire grains, and lean proteins, has been displayed to make a defensive difference.

Notwithstanding these dietary elements, there is an additional way-of-life factor that can add to the advancement of skin cancer.

One of the most significant is sun openness. Delayed openness to the sun's unsafe UV rays is one of the essential risk factors for skin cancer. Thus, it's critical to safeguard your skin from the sun by wearing a defensive dress and utilizing sunscreen with a high SPF rating.

Here are a few hints for you to eat to reduce your chances of getting Melanoma.

Load up on Vegetables: Leafy foods are wealthy in antioxidants, which can assist with shielding your skin from the harmful impacts of free extremists. Expect to eat various brilliant products of the soil consistently, including berries, citrus natural products, mixed greens, and cruciferous vegetables like broccoli and cauliflower.

Pick sound fats: Omega-3 unsaturated fats, which are found in greasy fish like salmon and fish, as well as nuts and seeds like chia seeds and flaxseeds, can assist with lessening aggravation in the body and may bring down your risk of skin cancer.

Keep away from handled and refined food sources: Handled and refined food varieties, like sweet bites and inexpensive food, have been connected to an expanded risk of skin cancer. All things being equal centers around entire food sources like entire grains, lean proteins, and new products of the soil.

Drink a lot of water: Remaining hydrated is significant for by and large wellbeing, and can likewise assist with keeping your skin solid and hydrated. Expect to drink no less than eight glasses of water a day, from there, the sky's the limit if you are dynamic or live in a blistering environment.

The possibility that skin cancer can be relieved by diet changes isn't demonstrated, or reasonable. Most regarded bodies do anyway concur on a basic level that similarly as with a few other cancers, the diet has a section to play.

There is restricted proof that the spread of mostly nonmelanoma skin cancers might be decreased by dietary elements. There is more beneficial proof that diet can have an impact in forestalling the beginning or repeat of skin cancer.

The Advantage Of Antioxidants

Rather than diet, skin cancer is mostly brought about by UV rays from the sun, or tanning machines. They help to create free extremists, unsound oxygen atoms which harm the DNA in skin cells, prompting changes and skin cancer.

A diet wealthy in antioxidants can assist with warding off free revolutionaries, diminishing harm. You could note we decided to say diet, rather than supplements. An enhancement is better than a kick in the pants than only proof recommends that antioxidants from food are more compelling:

Beta Carotene - A normally happening supplement, which converts to vitamin An inside your body. Predominant in orange-hued leafy foods, like apricot, mango, squash, carrots, or yams.

L-ascorbic acid - Acknowledged examinations have demonstrated L-ascorbic acid to be harmful to cancer cells, albeit again there is no proof of a healing impact. Oranges, lemons, limes, and strawberries are a decent source of verdant green vegetables.

Vitamin D - The skin creates vitamin D through openness to the sun, albeit over-openness isn't an advantage. A couple of cancer-opposing properties are acknowledged for vitamin D and safe sources incorporate cod liver oil, salmon, or more modest sums in dairy items.

Vitamin E - Demonstrated to have the impact you need on free revolutionaries and to assist the skin with going about as a defensive boundary. A positive instance of diet being superior to supplements, like almonds, or other nuts, sunflower seeds, spinach, or soya beans.

Lycopene - Made by development to shield tomatoes from sun harm and liable to do likewise for your skin. A red-hued antioxidant you will track down in tomatoes, watermelon, apricots, grapefruit, and blood oranges.

Omega-3 Unsaturated fats They are accepted to decrease aggravation and similarly, confine compound cycles that advance skin cancer. Greasy fish like salmon or mackerel are a decent source, alongside pecans and flax seeds.

Polyphenols - Strong antioxidants are most generally tracked down in tea.
They are again accepted to decrease aggravation and may repress cancer development. Newly prepared green tea is a decent source to pick, albeit dark tea is a fair choice.

Selenium - Beneficial examinations have demonstrated the way that an expanded admission of selenium can significantly affect a scope of cancers, including the skin. Brazil nuts are a respectable source to pick from, chicken is another supplier.

Zinc - An impetus that initiates antioxidants inside your body, assists the invulnerable framework with working great to fend off cancers, and diminishes DNA harm. A scope of meats offers zinc, close shellfish, and vegetables like chickpeas, beans, or lentils.

Eating For Wellbeing

There are various explanations behind a solid diet, including cancer counteraction.

Enhancements can in any case have a section to play, nicotinamide, a type of vitamin B3, is a demonstrated model. In a twofold visually impaired preliminary attempt by Sydney College, a 2 X 500mg everyday portion supposedly reduced the occurrence of new non-melanoma skin cancer by 20 to 30%.

At a sensible dose, perhaps with clinical counsel, other nutrient enhancements are superior to not supporting your body. We would in any case underline the benefits of dietary change.

Any assisted diet with canning given with skin cancer counteraction, or control is gladly received, similar to extra benefits.

The benefits of a reasonable, natural-centered diet are laid out and critical to a sound life.

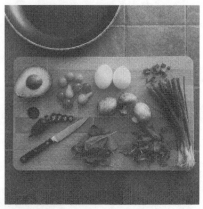

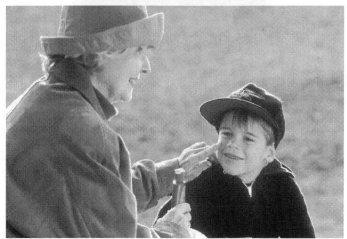

Chapter 1

Anti-Skin Cancer Foods and Their Benefits

While there are numerous therapies accessible for skin cancer, avoidance is dependably the best game plan. One method for forestalling skin cancer is by eating foods that are known to have anti-skin cancer properties. We will examine the absolute best anti-skin cancer foods and their benefits.

Berries

Berries are a gathering of natural products that are known for their high antioxidant content.

Antioxidants are substances that assist to safeguard the body from damage brought about by free extremists, which are unsound atoms that can cause cell damage and add to the advancement of cancer. Berries are particularly high in a kind of antioxidant called anthocyanins, which have been displayed to decrease the risk of developing skin cancer.

Notwithstanding their antioxidant content, berries are likewise high in L-ascorbic acid, which has been displayed to assist with shielding the skin from UV damage. The absolute best berries to eat for their anti-skin cancer properties incorporate blueberries, strawberries, raspberries, and blackberries.

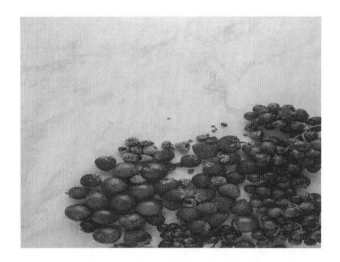

Vegetables

Vegetables are a superb wellspring of numerous supplements that are fundamental for good health, including nutrients A, C, and E, as well as folate and beta-carotene. These supplements have been displayed to have anti-cancer properties, and they can assist with safeguarding the skin from damage brought about by UV rays.

The absolute best leafy greens to eat for their anti-skin cancer properties incorporate spinach, kale, collard greens, and Swiss chard. These greens can be eaten raw in plates of mixed greens or cooked as a side dish.

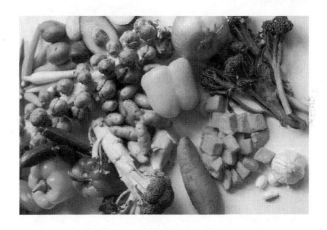

Tomatoes
Tomatoes are one more food that is known for its anti-cancer properties. Tomatoes are high in a substance called lycopene, which is a strong antioxidant that has been displayed to diminish the risk of developing a few kinds of cancer, including skin cancer.

Notwithstanding their lycopene content, tomatoes are additionally high in L-ascorbic acid, which as referenced prior, can assist with shielding the skin from UV damage. Tomatoes can be eaten raw in servings of mixed greens or cooked in sauces, soups, and stews.

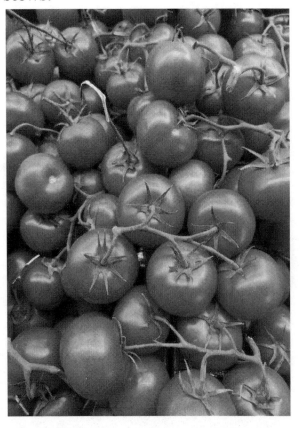

Green Tea

Green tea is a drink that is high in antioxidants known as catechins.

In a recent report, specialists found that green tea utilization prompted fewer growths instigated by UV light in mice. This was expected from a flavanol contained in both green and dark tea known as EGCG.

These antioxidants have been displayed to have anti-cancer properties and can assist with shielding the skin from UV damage. Notwithstanding its anti-skin cancer properties, green tea has likewise been displayed to have numerous other health benefits, including further developed heart health and weight loss.

Some many people have found out that concentrating on green tea found that it diminished skin damage from UVA light and safeguarded against the lessening of collagen. Collagen is our body's most plentiful protein. It gives skin its uprightness and immovability.

Taste this: Capitalize on summer produce and stir up some cooled green tea with ice, mint leaves, and your number one citrus natural products.

To get the most anti-skin cancer benefits from green tea, it is ideal to consistently drink it. One to three cups each day is suggested.

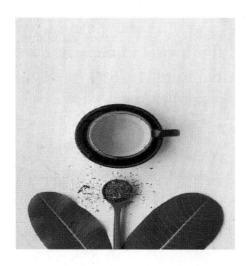

Fish

Fish is a great wellspring of omega-3 unsaturated fats, which have been displayed to have anti-cancer properties. Omega-3 unsaturated fats can assist with lessening irritation in the body, which can add to the advancement of cancer. Furthermore, a few examinations have demonstrated the way that omega-3 unsaturated fats can assist in decreasing the risk of developing skin cancer.

The absolute best fish to eat for their anti-skin cancer properties incorporate salmon, sardines, and mackerel. These fish are high in omega-3 unsaturated fats and can be barbecued, heated, or cooked.

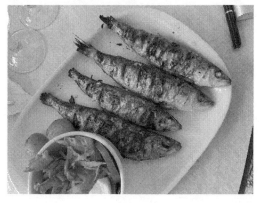

Blueberries

Blueberries are rich in strong antioxidants that ward off free extremists that can damage the skin because of sun openness and stress. Blueberries are much more impressive on the off chance that they're a wild assortment. They're likewise a generally excellent wellspring of L-ascorbic acid, which can assist with keeping wrinkles from a day near the ocean.

- **Fast breakfast:** Get your feast prep on within a quick breakfast parfait made with layers of natively constructed, 15-minute blueberry chia jam, coconut yogurt, and granola.

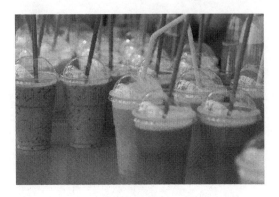

Watermelon

Tomatoes are known for containing lycopene, an antioxidant liable for tomatoes' red tone. However, watermelons contain undeniably more. Lycopene retains both UVA and UVB radiation, even though it might require half a month for the skin to turn out to be more photoprotective because of its turnover rate, as indicated by a recent report.

Following half a month of day-to-day, succulent watermelon utilization (not too difficult to even think about overseeing in the warm climate!), lycopene can ultimately go about as a characteristic sunblock. Analysts note, however, that it isn't guaranteed to replace other defensive measures, similar to SPF and sun-defensive attires, against sunspots and skin damage. Be that as it may, with regards to anti-maturing, this additional lift sure won't do any harm.

Nuts and seeds

Pecans, hemp seeds, chia seeds, and flax all contain omega-3 fundamental unsaturated fats. Fish and eggs are additionally extraordinary wellsprings of this spotless, skin-adoring fat. Our bodies can't make omega-3s, so it's fundamental that we get them from our eating regimen.

How do omega-3s help your skin? They assist with keeping up with your skin's respectability and are anti-provocative, as well. Omega-3s likewise help your body normally adapt to the impacts of investing excessively much energy in the sun.

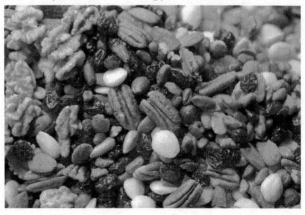

Cauliflower

With regards to veggies and organic products, an overall health rule to live and shop by is to incline toward more energetically hued eats. This is because they're probably going to have more antioxidants.

Yet, don't allow cauliflower's pale florets to trick you. This cruciferous veggie is the special case for the standard. Cauliflower contains powerful antioxidants that assist with warding off oxidative pressure from free extremists.

On top of this advantage, cauliflower is likewise a normally sun-defensive food because of histidine. This alpha-amino corrosive invigorates the development of urocanic corrosive, which assimilates UV radiation.

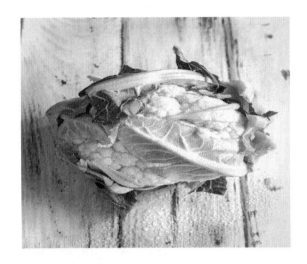

- **Barbecue this**: If you want to have breakfast, attempt a cauliflower steak with velvety bean stew lime sauce.

Super Summer Sunblock Smoothie

Who says you can't drink your sun shield? This smoothie assists you with beating the intensity and contains all of the skin-defensive ingredients recorded previously. Add it to your morning pivot for a healthier gleam the entire summer.

Ingredients

- ☐ 1 1/2 cups green tea, cooled
- ☐ 1 cup blueberries
- ☐ 1 cup watermelon
- ☐ 1/2 cup cauliflower
- ☐ 1 little carrot
- ☐ 2 tbsp. hemp hearts
- ☐ 1 tbsp. lemon juice
- ☐ 3-5 ice cubes

Directions

Place ingredients in a blender. Mix until smooth. For a thicker smoothie, utilize 1 cup of green tea.

While these supplement-rich, entire foods might uphold the health of your skin when presented with UV light, remember that they're not a substitute for sunscreen. Still, apply sunscreen consistently to forestall sun damage and skin cancer. Consider these foods some additional protection assuming you happen to over soak the sun's rays.

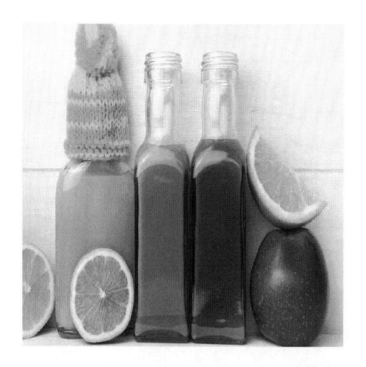

Super Summer Sunblock Smoothie

Chapter 2

Foods to Avoid and Superfoods that Help Prevent Skin Cancer

While prevention of skin cancer is troublesome, decreasing the risk of creating skin cancer by following a sound diet is conceivable. We will examine the foods to avoid and superfoods that help prevent skin cancer.

Foods to Avoid

Processed Foods

Processed foods are high in sugar, salt, and undesirable fats that can aggravate and harm the skin. These foods additionally contain synthetics and additives that can prompt DNA harm and increment the risk of skin cancer.

Fried Foods

Fried foods are high in unfortunate fats and oils that can aggravate and harm the skin. These foods likewise contain acrylamide, a substance that structures when foods are cooked at high temperatures and have been connected to an expanded risk of skin cancer.

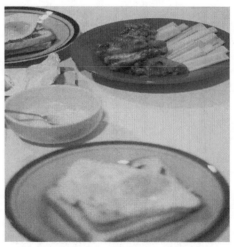

Alcohol

Over-the-top alcohol utilization can debilitate the invulnerable framework, prompting a higher risk of skin cancer. Alcohol additionally dries out the skin, making it more defenseless to harm from the sun's UV beams.

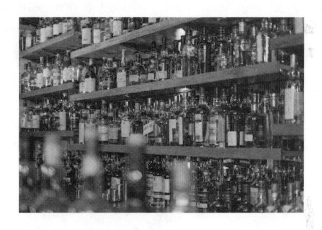

High-Glycemic Foods

High-glycemic foods will be foods that raise glucose levels rapidly, prompting irritation and harm to the skin. These foods incorporate white bread, pasta, and sweet tidbits.

Superfoods that Help Prevent Skin Cancer

Red foods are grown from the ground

Red foods grown from the ground are wealthy in lycopene, another cell reinforcement that might safeguard your skin against sun harm, as per a concentrate in the English Diary of Dermatology. Tomatoes, tomato sauce, watermelon, pink grapefruit, apricots, blood oranges, and papaya are great wellsprings of lycopene.

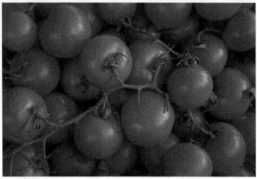

Vegetables

Additionally wealthy in zinc: Vegetables, which might improve your body's resistant framework and restore cell reinforcement levels. Add a sprinkle of beans, like chickpeas, dark beans, and edamame, to everything from servings of mixed greens or soups. Attempt bean plunges, for example, hummus with crude vegetables for a delish-and-nutrish nibble.

Orange foods are grown from the ground

Orange produce is plentiful in beta-carotene, which is switched over completely to vitamin A in your body. Going after orange products in the soil routinely may diminish the risk for certain cancers. Carrots, yams, apricots, melon, and squash are incredible wellsprings of beta-carotene. While research on the impact of beta carotene and melanoma is uncertain, some proof backings the job of vitamin A in diminishing the risk of creating melanoma, as per the Diary of Analytical Dermatology.

VitaminD invigorated foods

Research shows that satisfactory vitamin D admission is related to a diminished risk of melanoma and that individuals who are vitamin D insufficient have a less fortunate result when determined to have melanoma. Remember vitamin D invigorated foods for your eating regimens like milk, yogurt, oat, and juice.

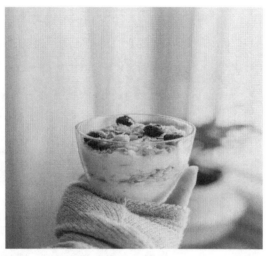

Citrus organic products

Citrus natural products are great wellsprings of L-ascorbic acid, which might offer some insurance from cancer-causing free revolutionaries. Nibble on oranges, and add a cut of new lemon or lime to a glass of water for an additional increase in L-ascorbic acid. However, not a citrus organic product, strawberries are rich in vitamin C too.

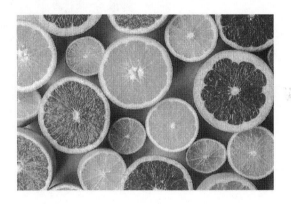

Tea

The polyphenols found in dark and green tea have been connected to an assortment of medical advantages, including cancer prevention. Research shows that green tea, explicitly, can hinder the development of melanoma cells. Have a go at adding some green tea (hot or chilled) to your everyday daily practice.

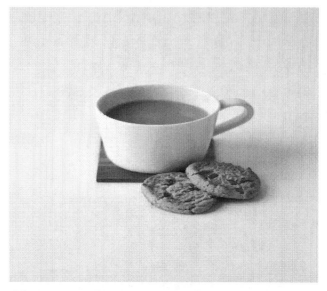

Coffee

On the off chance that you now drink coffee consistently like by far most Americans, you may as of now be receiving the counter skin cancer rewards of the refreshment without acknowledging it! If you don't drink coffee, you may be savvy to begin drinking it all the more consistently - particularly assuming you're getting your caffeine from sources like soft drinks.

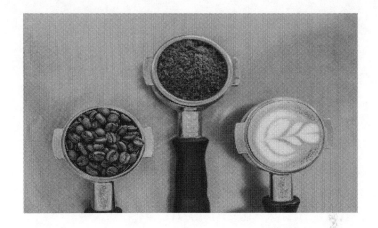

A review performed by scientists from Brigham and Ladies' Emergency Clinic and Harvard Clinical School tracked down a connection between expanded coffee consumption and a diminished risk of basal cell carcinoma, the most well-known type of skin cancer.

The scientists found that in addition to the fact that there was a connection between coffee utilization and diminished skin cancer risk, you could likewise bring down your risk significantly further by expanding your utilization.

While a solid eating routine can't prevent skin cancer, it can diminish the risk of fostering the sickness. By avoiding processed and fried foods, alcohol, and high-glycemic foods, and consolidating superfoods like berries, salad greens, tomatoes, nuts and seeds, and green tea, people can advance their skin well-being and diminish their risk of skin cancer.

It is likewise essential to make sure to wear sunscreen and a defensive dress and to avoid direct openness to the sun during top hours, especially on the off chance that one has a history of skin cancer or a family background of the infection.

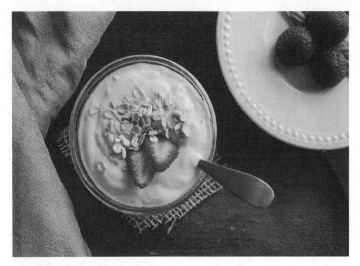

Yogurt Strawberries

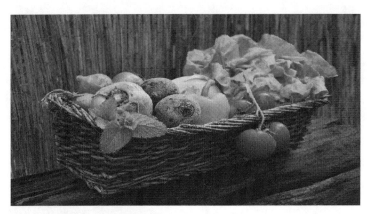

A Vegetable Basket

Chapter 3

Recipes for Breakfast that Promote Skin Health

There's something else to getting healthy, sparkling skin than purchasing the ideal skincare items. Even if you use all the concealer and makeup in the world, your skin will not look its best unless you eat a diet rich in beauty foods.

Make these breakfasts that improve beauty to kick off your day in the right way. They are packed with beautiful foods that keep your skin looking young, fresh, and radiant.

Omelet Italian-Style

Tomatoes add delicious flavor to this straightforward omelet, yet they likewise support skin well-being. Consuming these bright red vegetables may aid in the treatment of sunburn, increase collagen production, and even smooth skin.

PREP TIME: 5 min

COOK TIME: 9 minutes in total 14-minute

Ingredients:
- ☐ 1 Tbsp chopped onion
- ☐ 1 Tbsp chopped green bell pepper
- ☐ 1 Tbsp chopped tomatoes (plus additional tomatoes for garnish)
- ☐ 1 beaten egg
- ☐ 2 beaten egg whites
- ☐ 12 teaspoons Italian seasoning

☐ 1 Tbsp grated Parmesan cheese

Procedures

Step 1: ADD onions and peppers to a medium nonstick skillet covered with a cooking shower over medium intensity. Cook, occasionally stirring, for about 2 minutes, or until hot.

Step 2: Toss in the tomatoes. Cook for around a brief length, or until simply beginning to mellow.

Step 3: Include egg yolks and whites. Season with salt and pepper. Cook on low heat for about 5 minutes, or until the bottom is set, by lifting the cooked edges of the egg mixture with a fork so the uncooked egg can run underneath. Cook the eggs until they are set, about one to two minutes.

Step 4: SPRINKLE with the cheddar and overlap the omelet fifty.

Greek-Style Frittata

Contains 217 calories, 2 grams of fat, 0.5 grams of saturated fat, 79 milligrams of sodium, 49 grams of carbohydrates, 26 grams of sugar, 5 grams of fiber, 4.5 grams of protein Greek-Style Frittata: This mouthwatering morning meal packs a big beauty punch. The spinach's vitamin A stimulates cell turnover, giving you that desired glow. Eggs with a lot of protein help make collagen, which makes your skin more elastic, and they also give you more of the antioxidants lutein and zeaxanthin, which protect your skin from UV damage.

PREP TIME: 10 minutes to cook

COOK TIME: 20 mins

SERVINGS: 30 minutes

Ingredients

- ☐ 4 eggs
- ☐ 12 crumbled feta cheese
- ☐ 12 sliced grape tomatoes
- ☐ 1 Tbsp olive oil
- ☐ 14 nonfat milk
- ☐ 1 tsp oregano
- ☐ spinach leaves
- ☐ frozen diced potatoes
- ☐ onions, and peppers (found in bags in the freezer section)

1. LOWLY PREHEAT the broiler. In the meantime, heat a medium skillet on low. Cover the spinach with a lid for one minute, or until it has barely wilted. Put everything in a small bowl and set it aside. Clean the pan.

2. Heat olive oil in a cleaned skillet on medium. Cover and cook, turning occasionally, until the potato mixture is tender but firm (5 to 7 minutes). Place aside.

3. Combine the milk and eggs in a medium bowl. To taste, add oregano, cheese, tomatoes, spinach, and salt and pepper.

4. Place a nonstick ovenproof skillet of 8 to 10 inches over low heat and spray it with cooking spray. Cover base equally with potatoes and pour egg blend up and over. Cook the eggs until they are set, about ten minutes. To cook the top of the frittata, place the skillet under the broiler for one to two minutes.

Sustenance (per serving) 206 cal, 12 g fat, 4 g sat fat, 343 mg sodium, 13 g carb, 2 g sugar, 2.5 g fiber, 12 g protein.

Strawberry-Kiwi Smoothie

Strawberry and kiwi provide a significant amount of skin-smoothing vitamin C in this 5-minute smoothie. According to Drayer, vitamin C helps collagen synthesis and prevents wrinkles. That's a welcome change!

PREP TIME: 5 minutes to cook

Total Time: 0 minutes

SERVINGS: 5 minutes

Ingredients
- ☐ 4 cups cold apple juice
- ☐ 1 ripe banana, sliced
- ☐ 1 kiwifruit, sliced
- ☐ 5 frozen strawberries
- ☐ 12 teaspoon honey

Blend the juice, banana, kiwifruit, and strawberries. Blend until it is smooth.

Nutritional Information (per Serving): 87 calories, 0.5 grams of fat, 0 grams of saturated fat, 4 milligrams of sodium, 22 grams of carbohydrates, 17 grams of sugar, 1.5 grams of fiber, 0.5 grams of protein.

Walnut Protein Pancakes

These hearty pancakes contain whole grains, protein, and a little bit of fat—the ideal components for a healthy breakfast. However, they also contain a few tablespoons of walnuts, which are a good source of the ALA omega-3 fatty acids that are beneficial to the health of the skin. We are aware that we may experience dry, scaly skin if our diet lacks ALA.

PREP TIME: 6 minutes to cook
Ingredients
- ☐ 1 cup quick-cooking oats
- ☐ 12 cups whole grain pastry flour
- ☐ 2 tablespoons chopped walnuts
- ☐ 12 teaspoons and pure foods featherweight baking powder
- ☐ 1 teaspoon ground cinnamon
- ☐ 1 scoop vanilla whey protein powder

☐ 3 egg whites

☐ 1 teaspoon pure vanilla extract

☐ 12 teaspoons fat-free ricotta cheese

☐ 34 teaspoons fat-free milk

1. Apply cooking spray to a nonstick skillet, wipe off any excess with a paper towel, and then set the towel aside. Between pancakes, wipe the skillet with this towel to remove any crumbs from the pancake batter and recoat it with oil.

2. The skillet should be preheated to medium-low before being turned down to low.

3. Consolidate the dry fixings in a bowl and blend well. After that, incorporate the wet ingredients.

4. In the skillet, spoon about 12 cups of the batter in. Cook until firm and golden brown, about one to two minutes. Cook the pancake on the

other side for another 30 seconds to 1 minute, or until it is golden brown. Place the pancake on a serving plate. Wipe the skillet with a paper towel.

5. Make eight pancakes by repeating Step 4 with the remaining batter.

Pro Tip: To ensure that the pancakes cook evenly, it is essential to cook them over low heat. Assuming the intensity is too high, the exterior will consume while the inner parts stay runny.

Lean Tip: Restrict yourself to 3 hotcakes for each sitting and store the rest in the ice chest.

Per serving, there are 351 calories, 7 grams of fat, 1 gram of saturated fat, 155 milligrams of sodium, 46 grams of carbohydrates, 8 grams of sugar, 6 grams of fiber, and 24 grams of protein.

Banana Split Biscuits

You'll partake in every single piece of these shockingly light breakfast biscuits while getting your skin some hydrating dark chocolate. Concentrates show that beneficial mixtures in dark chocolate increment skin hydration and diminish scaling. In any case, it prescribes adhering to a 1-ounce serving, making sense that a lot of sugar is solid.

Planning TIME: 7 min

COOK TIME: 13 min

All out TIME: 20 min

SERVINGS: 12

Ingredients

- ☐ 1½ c walnuts coarsely slashed
- ☐ 1½ c regular baking flour
- ☐ ¾ c semisweet chocolate smaller than expected baking chips
- ☐ 1 Tbsp baking powder

- ☐ ½ tsp ground cinnamon
- ☐ ½ tsp salt
- ☐ ½ c pressed dull earthy colored sugar
- ☐ ¼ c canola oil
- ☐ ¼ c fat-free plain Greek yogurt
- ☐ ¼ c fat-free milk
- ☐ 1 egg
- ☐ 1 exceptionally ready banana, pounded (about ⅓ c)
- ☐ 1 tsp vanilla concentrate

1. PREHEAT the oven to 375°F. Cover a 12-cup biscuit tin with a cooking splash.

2. MEASURE ½ cup of the walnuts into a food processor and drudgery to a fine feast. Place the ground walnuts, flour, chocolate chips, baking powder, cinnamon, and salt in an enormous bowl and mix until completely consolidated.

3. Join the earthy-colored sugar, oil, yogurt, milk, egg, banana, and vanilla concentrate in a medium bowl and mix until smooth. Add the banana blend to the flour combination and mix until completely joined. Mix in the leftover 1 cup walnuts and blend well (the player will be thick).

4. FILL the biscuit cups three-fourths full and prepare for 13 to 15 minutes, or until the tops spring back softly when contacted. Eliminate the biscuits from the container and let them cool on a rack. Tip: This player is extremely thick, similar to the treat mixture, so have a go at utilizing a frozen yogurt scoop to fill the tins rapidly and without any problem.

Tip: Make it a Level Tummy dinner by serving it with 1 pear (103 calories). Absolute dinner: 390 calories

Nourishment (per serving) 287 cal, 16.5 g fat, 3 g sat fat, 234 mg sodium, 33 g carb, 17 g sugar, 2 g fiber, 5 g protein.

Bagels with Lox and Cream Cheddar

One explanation your skin begins to look dull as you become older is because it creates fewer oils. She suggests getting your shine back by adding some omega-3 unsaturated fats into your diet. Salmon is one of the most mind-blowing wellsprings of omega-3s, however, it's not necessarily in all cases breakfast amicable. Give smoked salmon a shot in your bagel to add a little exquisite flavor.

Planning TIME: 10 min

COOK TIME: 0 min

Complete: 10 min

SERVINGS: 4

Ingredients

- ☐ 6 oz fat-free cream cheddar, at room temperature
- ☐ 2 Tbsp hacked new dill
- ☐ 2 tsp depleted tricks, slashed
- ☐ 4 pumpernickel bagels, split
- ☐ 3 oz smoked salmon
- ☐ ½ sm red onion, daintily cut
- ☐ ⅓ English cucumber, cut
- ☐ 1 tomato, cut into 8 slim cuts
- ☐ 4 leaves lettuce

Join the cream cheddar, dill, and tricks in a little bowl. Spread 4 bagel parts with 1 tablespoon of the cream-cheddar blend. Top with layers of salmon, onion, cucumber, tomato, and lettuce. Cover with the leftover bagel parts. Slice each sandwich down the middle.

Lemon-Mustard Dill Spread

The kinds of salmon and dill have forever been an exemplary match. For a simple to-make-ahead backup to this sandwich, in a little bowl, join;

- ☐ ⅓ cup low-fat mayonnaise
- ☐ 2 tablespoons hacked new dill
- ☐ 1 tablespoon slashed new parsley
- ☐ 2 teaspoons Dijon mustard
- ☐ 1 teaspoon lemon juice
- ☐ ½ teaspoon ground lemon strip
- ☐ ground dark pepper to taste

Nourishment (per serving) 386 cal, 4 g fat, 0.5 g sat fat, 835 mg sodium, 67 g carb, 12 g sugar, 5 g fiber, 23 g protein

Green Tea, Blueberry, and Banana Smoothie

Green tea is as of now known as a marvel drink that forestalls coronary illness and perhaps amps up digestion, yet presently you can add "excellence sponsor" to its rundown of benefits. Studies have shown that drinking green tea preceding going out in the sun might assist with diminishing harm from UV rays, and its strong cell reinforcements may likewise give assurance against skin cancer. Blending in blueberries additionally expands the cell reinforcement force of this smoothie. A new report found that ellagic corrosiveness in blueberries may forestall skin harm.

Planning TIME: 5 min

COOK TIME: 0 min

Complete TIME: 5 min

SERVINGS: 1

Ingredients

- ☐ 3 Tbsp water
- ☐ 1 green tea sack
- ☐ 2 tsp honey
- ☐ 1½ c frozen blueberries
- ☐ ½ drug banana
- ☐ ¾ c calcium-strengthened light vanilla soy milk

1. MICROWAVE water on high until steaming hot in a little glass estimating cup or bowl. Add the tea pack and let it brew for 3 minutes. Eliminate the tea sack. Mix honey into tea until it breaks down.

2. Consolidate berries, bananas, and milk in a blender with ice squashing capacity.

3. ADD tea to the blender. Mix fixings on ice pound or most noteworthy setting until smooth. (A few blenders might require extra water to handle the combination.) Empty the smoothie into a tall glass and serve

Recipe tips: Whenever put away for a few hours in a Canteen, shake vivaciously before pouring. The smoothie will be delectable however more slender than when newly made.

Nourishment (per serving) 269 cal, 2.5 g fat, 0 g sat fat, 52 mg sodium, 63 g carb, 39 g sugar, 8 g fiber, 4 g protein.

Entire Grain Cereal and a Banana

However, cereal and organic products might appear as a fundamental breakfast, but the benefits of this dinner are everything except conventional. Entire grains are stuffed with cell reinforcements, which are the vital fixings to a young coloring. A few cereals, similar to Add Up, are braced with zinc, which has a major stunner benefit. "Zinc is nature's calming mineral. It's fundamental for building sound collagen.

Planning TIME: 3 min

COOK TIME: 6 min

All out TIME: 9 min

SERVINGS: 1

Ingredients

- ☐ ¾ c entire grain drops of cereal
- ☐ 1 sm banana, cut
- ☐ 2 tsp slashed walnuts
- ☐ 1 c fat-free milk
- ☐ 3 oz prepared turkey breakfast frankfurter

Join the cereal, banana, walnuts, and milk in a bowl. Present with the frankfurter.

Nourishment (per serving) 399 cal, 5.5 g fat, 0.5 g sat fat, 472 mg sodium, 61 g carb, 29 g sugar, 9 g fiber, 34 g protein.

Sweet Potato Pancakes

Sweet potatoes have that magnificent sweet flavor, and they're loaded with skin-safeguarding advantages. Beta-carotene in sweet potatoes resembles palatable sunscreen. Consuming carotenoids like beta-carotene is related to less burn from the sun, and they're changed over completely to vitamin A, which keeps your skin delicate and smooth.

These little snacks are ideally suited for an end-of-the-week informal breakfast presented with hostile to maturing berries.

Planning TIME: 15 min

COOK TIME: 15 min

All out TIME: 30 min

SERVINGS: 12

Ingredients

- ☐ 12 oz sweet potato, peeled and shredded
- ☐ 12 oz chestnut potato, peeled and shredded
- ☐ 1 prescription onion, ground, abundance liquid squeezed out
- ☐ 1 egg
- ☐ ¼ c entire wheat flour
- ☐ ½ tsp salt
- ☐ ¼ tsp ground dark pepper
- ☐ 3 Tbsp olive oil
- ☐ ¼ c light harsh cream

☐ ¼ c low-fat mayonnaise
☐ ¼ c finely slashed apple
☐ 1 Tbsp arranged horseradish, squeezed dry

1. PREHEAT the oven to 200°F.

2. Join the sweet potato, chestnut potato, onion, egg, flour, salt, and pepper. Structure the combination into 24 patties, around 2 tablespoons each and around 1½ creeps in diameter.

3. HEAT 2 tablespoons of the oil in an enormous nonstick skillet over medium intensity. Add 12 pancakes and cook, turning once, for 7 minutes, or until brilliant and cooked through. Move to a baking sheet and keep warm in the oven. Heat the excess 1 tablespoon oil and rehash.

4. In the meantime, in a little bowl, consolidate the sharp cream, mayonnaise, apple, and horseradish; blend well. Present with the pancakes.

Sustenance (per serving) 118 cal, 6 g fat, 1 g sat fat, 166 mg sodium, 14 g carb, 3 g sugar, 2 g fiber, 2 g protein.

Lovely Berry Smoothie

Containing anthocyanins (strong cancer prevention agents that assist to safeguard the skin from free revolutionaries), and loaded with L-ascorbic acid, blueberries can assist with advancing the creation of collagen - keeping your skin firm! The blueberry has been distinguished as containing the most cell reinforcements per serving of any organic product.

Grapefruit

Vitamin C in grapefruit aids in the repair of damage to the skin caused by free radicals such as those produced by the sun and pollutants when consumed fresh. It makes more collagen, which makes new skin grow, lessens wrinkles, and makes the skin feel smoother overall. Containing lycopene (subsequently the red tone), grapefruit is likewise perfect for decreasing aggravation of the skin and redness.

Spinach
Alpha lipoic acids (ALA) are abundant in spinach and other green leafy vegetables. ALA is one of the most impressive enemies of maturing specialists that anyone could hope to find. It additionally goes about as a calming, diminishing under-eye circle, puffiness, redness, and blotches while limiting the presence of kinks.

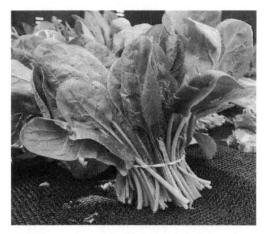

<u>Turmeric</u>

Germ-free and antibacterial, turmeric not just assists with clearing skin break-out scars and irritation yet additionally diminishes oil discharge by sebaceous organs. Because it aids in the prevention of melanoma, it is ideal for use in the preparation of breakfast and meals.

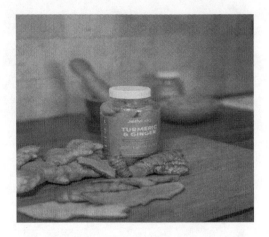

<u>Salmon</u>

Wealthy in Omega 3 unsaturated fats that support the skin by lessening the body's development of provocative substances, diminishing stopped-up pores. Salmon has a lot of dimethylaminoethanol, which protects cell membranes from the deterioration that causes premature aging and helps to strengthen them. Arachidonic acid production, which contributes to the formation of wrinkles and sagging of the skin, can also be reduced by DMAE.

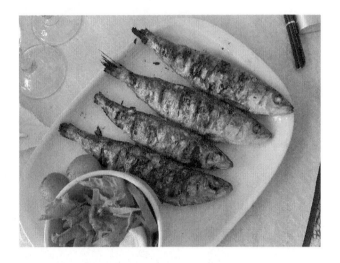

Fruit with oatmeal

Fiber and antioxidants from oats are excellent skin-nourishing nutrients. For more vitamins and minerals, add some fresh fruit like blueberries, strawberries, or sliced bananas.

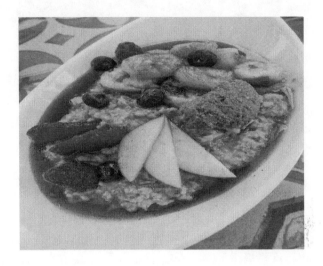

<u>Honeyed Greek yogurt with nuts</u>

Probiotics, which can help maintain healthy gut flora and improve skin health, can be found in Greek yogurt, making it an excellent source of protein. For some healthy fats and crunch, drizzle some honey over the dish and add a few nuts like almonds or walnuts.

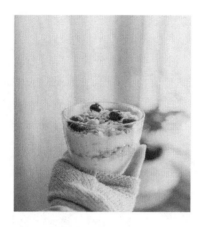

<u>Toast with avocado</u>

Avocado is plentiful in solid fats and nutrients E and C, which can assist with keeping your skin hydrated and sound. On whole grain toast, spread mashed avocado and season with salt and pepper. For more protein, you can also add smoked salmon or a poached egg.

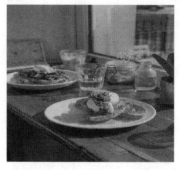

Bowl of smoothies

For a breakfast packed with nutrients, combine some frozen fruit like mango or berries with Greek yogurt, almond milk, and a handful of spinach or kale. Top with some granola, nuts, or coconut pieces for some crunch.

Breakfast bowl with quinoa

For a filling and nutritious breakfast, cook quinoa in almond milk and add cinnamon, chopped nuts, and dried fruit like raisins or apricots. Cinnamon can help regulate blood sugar levels and reduce inflammation, and quinoa is a great source of protein and fiber.

Keep in mind that eating a healthy breakfast is only one part of living a healthy life. To keep your skin looking its best, make sure to drink plenty of water, get enough sleep, and avoid smoking and drinking too much alcohol.

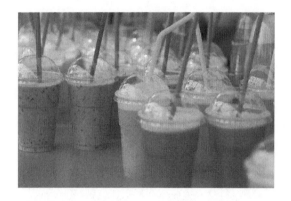

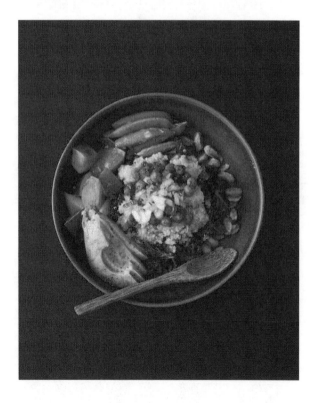

Chapter 4

<u>Salads and Appetizers to Boost Your Immune System</u>

Eating a healthy and adjusted diet is critical for keeping major areas of strength for a system. Salads and Appetizers are incredible choices for boosting your immune system since they are frequently loaded with nutrients, minerals, and antioxidants that assist with supporting immune capability. We will investigate a few scrumptious and nutritious salads and tidbits that are not difficult to make and can assist with keeping your immune system solid.

Beet and Goat Cheese Salad

Beets are loaded with nutrients and minerals that can assist with supporting immune capability. They are high in L-ascorbic acid, folate, and manganese, which are exceedingly significant supplements for immune well-being. Goat cheese is likewise an incredible wellspring of immune-boosting supplements, including zinc and selenium.

Fixings:

- ☐ 4 medium beets, cooked and diced
- ☐ 4 ounces of disintegrated goat cheese
- ☐ 2 tablespoons cleaved new parsley
- ☐ 2 tablespoons slashed new chives
- ☐ 2 tablespoons olive oil
- ☐ 1 tablespoon apple juice vinegar
- ☐ Salt and pepper to taste

Directions

In a huge bowl, join the beets, goat cheese, parsley, and chives.

In a little bowl, whisk together the olive oil, apple juice vinegar, salt, and pepper.

Pour the dressing over the salad and toss to cover.

Serve chilled.

Avocado and Tomato Salad

Avocado is an extraordinary wellspring of healthy fats and antioxidants, while tomatoes are high in L-ascorbic acid and lycopene, which can assist with supporting immune capability.

Fixings:

2 avocados, diced
2 cups cherry tomatoes, halved
1/4 cup slashed new cilantro
1/4 cup slashed red onion
2 tablespoons lime juice
Salt and pepper to taste

Guidelines

In an enormous bowl, join the avocados, tomatoes, cilantro, and red onion.

Sprinkle the lime juice over the salad and season with salt and pepper to taste.

Toss to consolidate and serve chilled.

Broccoli and Quinoa Salad

Broccoli is plentiful in L-ascorbic acid, vitamin A, and fiber, which can all assist with supporting immune capability. Quinoa is likewise an extraordinary wellspring of protein and fiber, making it a filling and nutritious expansion to any salad.

Fixings
- ☐ 2 cups cooked quinoa
- ☐ 2 cups broccoli florets, steamed
- ☐ 1/4 cup hacked red onion
- ☐ 1/4 cup hacked new parsley
- ☐ 1/4 cup hacked new mint
- ☐ 2 tablespoons olive oil
- ☐ 1 tablespoon lemon juice
- ☐ Salt and pepper to taste

Guidelines

In an enormous bowl, consolidate the quinoa, broccoli, red onion, parsley, and mint.

In a little bowl, whisk together the olive oil, lemon squeeze, salt, and pepper.

Pour the dressing over the salad and toss to cover.

Serve chilled.

Carrot Ginger Soup

Carrots are an incredible wellspring of vitamin A, which can assist with supporting immune capability. Ginger is likewise powerful in mitigating and cell reinforcement, making it an extraordinary expansion to any immune-boosting recipe.

Fixings:

- ☐ 6 huge carrots, stripped and slashed
- ☐ 1 little onion, cleaved

- ☐ 1 tablespoon ground new ginger
- ☐ 2 cloves garlic, minced
- ☐ 4 cups vegetable stock
- ☐ 1/2 cup coconut milk
- ☐ Salt and pepper to taste

Guidelines

In an enormous pot, sauté the carrots, onion, ginger, and garlic in a touch of olive oil until the vegetables are delicate.

Add the vegetable stock and heat to the point of boiling.

Diminish the intensity and let the soup stew for 20-30

Greek Salad

Greek salad is an invigorating and supplement stuffed dish that is ideally suited for any season. It is made with new vegetables and spices, feta cheese, and a tart dressing. The blend of fixings in this salad gives an overflow of nutrients and minerals, including nutrients A, C, and K, calcium, and iron.

Fixings
- ☐ 1 head of romaine lettuce, slashed
- ☐ 1 cucumber, sliced
- ☐ 1 red onion, meagerly sliced
- ☐ 1 ringer pepper, daintily sliced
- ☐ 1 16 ounce of cherry tomatoes, halved
- ☐ 1/2 cup of disintegrated feta cheese
- ☐ 1/4 cup of Kalamata olives
- ☐ 1/4 cup of hacked new parsley
- ☐ 1/4 cup of hacked new dill
- ☐ 1/4 cup of olive oil
- ☐ 2 tablespoons of red wine vinegar
- ☐ 1 tablespoon of lemon juice
- ☐ 1 clove of garlic, minced
- ☐ Salt and pepper to taste

Guidelines
In an enormous bowl, consolidate the slashed lettuce, sliced cucumber, sliced red

onion, sliced chime pepper, and halved cherry tomatoes.

Add the disintegrated feta cheese, Kalamata olives, slashed parsley, and hacked dill.

In a little bowl, whisk together the olive oil, red wine vinegar, lemon juice, minced garlic, salt, and pepper.

Pour the dressing over the salad and toss to consolidate.

Serve right away.

Quinoa Salad

Quinoa is a superfood that is loaded with protein, fiber, fundamental nutrients, and minerals. It is an incredible base for a salad and can be joined with different vegetables and spices for a delectable and healthy dinner.

Fixings

- ☐ 1 cup of quinoa, flushed
- ☐ 2 cups of water

☐ 1 red ringer pepper, diced
☐ 1 yellow ringer pepper, diced
☐ 1 cucumber, diced
☐ 1/4 cup of slashed new parsley
☐ 1/4 cup of slashed new mint
☐ 1/4 cup of olive oil
☐ 2 tablespoons of red wine vinegar
☐ 1 tablespoon of honey
☐ Salt and pepper to taste

Guidelines

In a medium pan, join the quinoa and water.

Heat to the point of boiling, then, at that point, decrease the intensity to low and stew for 15-20 minutes, or until the quinoa is delicate and the water has been consumed.

Cushion the quinoa with a fork and move to a huge bowl.

Add the diced red and yellow ringer peppers, diced cucumber, cleaved parsley, and slashed mint.

In a little bowl, whisk together the olive oil, red wine vinegar, honey, salt, and pepper.

Pour the dressing over the salad and toss to join.

Serve right away.

Beet and Orange Salad

Beets are an extraordinary wellspring of antioxidants and L-ascorbic acid, while oranges are plentiful in L-ascorbic acid and different supplements. This salad is an extraordinary method for getting various supplements and flavors in a single dish.

Fixings

- ☐ 4 medium beets, cooked and sliced
- ☐ 2 oranges, stripped and sliced
- ☐ 1/4 cup of cleaved New mint
- ☐ 1/4 cup of cleaved new

Directions

Preheat the broiler to 375°F.

Envelop every beet with foil and put it on a baking sheet.

Cook in the broiler for 45-an hours, or until the beets are delicate.

Eliminate the broiler and let cool for a couple of moments.

Strip the beets and cut them into adjustments.

Orchestrate the best cuts and orange cuts on a serving platter.

Sprinkle with cleaved new mint.

Serve right away.

Tomato and Mozzarella Salad

Tomatoes are plentiful in antioxidants and L-ascorbic acid, while mozzarella cheese gives calcium and protein. This salad is an exemplary dish that is ideal for a light lunch or supper.

Fixings

- ☐ 4 medium tomatoes, sliced
- ☐ 8 ounces of new mozzarella cheese, sliced
- ☐ 1/4 cup of hacked new basil
- ☐ 1/4 cup of olive oil
- ☐ 2 tablespoons of balsamic vinegar
- ☐ Salt and pepper to taste

Guidelines

Organize the tomato cuts and mozzarella cheese cuts on a serving platter.

Sprinkle with slashed new basil.

In a little bowl, whisk together the olive oil, balsamic vinegar, salt, and pepper.

Sprinkle the dressing over the salad.

Serve right away.

Spinach and Strawberry Salad

Spinach is rich in iron and other fundamental nutrients and minerals, while strawberries are an extraordinary wellspring of L-ascorbic acid and cell reinforcements. This salad is an extraordinary method for getting various supplements and flavors in a single dish.

Fixings

- ☐ 4 cups of child spinach
- ☐ 2 cups of cut strawberries
- ☐ 1/4 cup of chopped pecans
- ☐ 1/4 cup of disintegrated feta cheese
- ☐ 1/4 cup of olive oil
- ☐ 2 tablespoons of balsamic vinegar
- ☐ 1 tablespoon of honey
- ☐ Salt and pepper to taste

Directions

In a huge bowl, consolidate the child spinach, cut strawberries, chopped pecans, and disintegrated feta cheese.

In a little bowl, whisk together the olive oil, balsamic vinegar, honey, salt, and pepper.

Pour the dressing over the plate of mixed greens and throw it to consolidate.

Serve right away.

Avocado Toast

Avocado toast is a straightforward and delightful appetizer that is loaded with healthy fats, fiber, and fundamental nutrients and minerals.

Fixings

- ☐ 2 cups of whole wheat bread, toasted
- ☐ 1 ready avocado, mashed
- ☐ 1/2 teaspoon of red pepper pieces
- ☐ Salt and pepper to taste

Directions

Spread the mashed avocado on the toasted bread cuts.

Sprinkle with red pepper pieces, salt, and pepper.

Serve right away.

Hummus and Veggie Platter

Hummus is a healthy dip that is produced using chickpeas and tahini. It is an incredible wellspring of protein, fiber, fundamental nutrients, and minerals. Match it with various fresh veggies for a delightful and healthy appetizer.

Fixings

- ☐ 1 cup of hummus
- ☐ 1 red chile pepper, cut
- ☐ 1 yellow chime pepper, cut
- ☐ 1 cucumber, cut
- ☐ 1 carrot, cut
- ☐ 1 celery stem, cut

Directions

Orchestrate the hummus and cut veggies on a platter.

Serve right away.

Roasted Garlic and White Bean Dip

White beans are an extraordinary wellspring of protein and fiber, while roasted garlic gives a scrumptious flavor and smell. This dip is a healthy and delectable appetizer that can be delighted with fresh veggies or whole grain saltines.

Fixings

- ☐ 1 head of garlic
- ☐ 1 jar of white beans, depleted and flushed
- ☐ 1/4 cup of olive oil
- ☐ 2 tablespoons of lemon juice
- ☐ 1/4 teaspoon of paprika
- ☐ Salt and pepper to taste

Directions

Preheat the stove to 400°F.

Remove the top of the head of garlic and put it on a piece of foil.

Sprinkle with olive oil and fold the foil over the garlic.

Broil on the stove for 30-40 minutes, or until the garlic is delicate and caramelized.

Eliminate from the stove and let cool for a couple of moments.

Get the roasted garlic cloves into a food processor or blender.

Add the white beans, olive oil, lemon juice, paprika, salt, and pepper.

Mix until smooth and velvety.

Serve right away.

Caprese Skewers

Caprese skewers are a straightforward and delectable appetizer that highlights fresh mozzarella cheese, cherry tomatoes, and basil. This dish is an extraordinary method for partaking in the kinds of an exemplary

Caprese salad in tomfoolery and simple to-eat design.

Fixings

- ☐ 8 ounces of fresh mozzarella cheese, cut into reduced-down pieces
- ☐ 1 16 ounce of cherry tomatoes
- ☐ Fresh basil leaves
- ☐ Balsamic coating
- ☐ Salt and pepper to taste

Directions

Thread the mozzarella cheese, cherry tomatoes, and basil leaves onto skewers.

Shower with balsamic coating and sprinkle with salt and pepper.

Serve right away.

Sweet Potato Fries

Sweet potatoes are an incredible wellspring of nutrients and minerals, including vitamin A, L-ascorbic acid, and potassium. These prepared sweet potato fries are a healthy and scrumptious option in contrast to customary french fries.

Fixings

- ☐ 2 medium sweet potatoes, cut into fries
- ☐ 2 tablespoons of olive oil
- ☐ 1 teaspoon of garlic powder
- ☐ 1/2 teaspoon of smoked paprika
- ☐ Salt and pepper to taste

Guidelines

Preheat the broiler to 425°F.

In an enormous bowl, throw the sweet potato fries with olive oil, garlic powder, smoked paprika, salt, and pepper.

Spread the sweet potato fries out in a solitary layer on a baking sheet.

Heat in the broiler for 20-25 minutes, or until the fries are firm and delicate.

Serve right away.

Sweet Potato Chips with Avocado Dip

Here's a recipe for Sweet Potato Chips with Avocado Dip that will make a scrumptious and healthy diet!

Sweet Potato Chips Fixings

- ☐ 2 enormous sweet potatoes
- ☐ 2 tbsp. of olive oil
- ☐ 1 tsp. of paprika
- ☐ 1 tsp. of garlic powder
- ☐ Salt and pepper to taste

Avocado Dip Fixings

- ☐ 2 ready avocados
- ☐ 1 lime, squeezed
- ☐ 1/4 cup of plain Greek yogurt
- ☐ 1 garlic clove, minced
- ☐ Salt and pepper to taste

Guidelines

Preheat the broiler to 400°F (200°C).

Strip and cut the sweet potatoes into thin, even cuts. You can utilize a mandoline or a sharp blade to do this.

In an enormous bowl, blend the sweet potato cuts with the olive oil, paprika, garlic powder, salt, and pepper until they are equitably covered.

Spread the sweet potato cuts in a solitary layer on a baking sheet fixed with parchment paper.

Heat the sweet potato cuts for 15-20 minutes, flipping them halfway through, until they are fresh and brilliant brown.

While the sweet potato chips are heating up, set up the avocado dip. Slice the avocados down the middle, eliminate the pit, and scoop the flesh into a medium-sized bowl.

Mash the avocado with a fork until it is smooth yet at the same time slightly chunky.

Add the lime juice, Greek yogurt, minced garlic, salt, and pepper to the bowl and mix until everything is all around consolidated.

Taste the avocado dip and change the flavoring on a case-by-case basis.

Serve the sweet potato chips warm with the avocado dip as dessert, Enjoy!

Edamame Hummus
Fixings
- ☐ 2 cups shelled edamame
- ☐ 1/4 cup tahini
- ☐ 1/4 cup olive oil
- ☐ 3 cloves garlic, minced
- ☐ 2 tablespoons lemon juice
- ☐ 1/2 teaspoon cumin
- ☐ 1/2 teaspoon salt
- ☐ 1/4 teaspoon dark pepper
- ☐ 2-3 tablespoons water

Discretionary fixings: paprika, chopped fresh parsley

Directions

Start by heating a pot of water in the oven. When bubbling, add the edamame and let cook for 4-5 minutes, until delicate. Channel the edamame and wash with cold water to cool.

In a food processor, add the cooked edamame, tahini, olive oil, minced garlic, lemon juice, cumin, salt, and dark pepper. Beat the combination until it's all around joined.

Add 2-3 tablespoons of water to the combination to thin it out and help it mix more smoothly. Keep on beating until the hummus reaches your ideal consistency. On the off chance that you favor a smoother hummus, you can keep it a tad longer.

When the hummus is prepared, move it to a serving bowl. Garnish with a sprinkle of paprika and chopped fresh parsley, whenever wanted.

Serve the edamame hummus with pita chips, saltines, or fresh vegetables for dipping.

Enjoy your heavenly and healthy edamame hummus!

Grilled Pineapple Skewers

Grilled pineapple skewers are a heavenly and healthy treat that's ideal for any event, from lawn barbecues to picnics in the recreation area. Here's a recipe that will help you make the ideal grilled pineapple skewers like clockwork.

Fixings

- ☐ 1 fresh pineapple
- ☐ 1/4 cup honey
- ☐ 1/4 cup squeezed orange
- ☐ 2 tablespoons lime juice
- ☐ 2 tablespoons earthy-colored sugar
- ☐ 1/2 teaspoon cinnamon
- ☐ 1/4 teaspoon nutmeg

Wooden skewers, absorbs water for 30 minutes

Directions

Preheat your barbecue to medium-high heat.

Remove the top and lower part of the pineapple, and then cut off the skin utilizing a sharp blade. Slice the pineapple down the middle lengthwise, and then cut each half into quarters.

Remove the tough center of each pineapple quarter and dispose of it. Cut the pineapple into 1-inch chunks.

In a little bowl, combine as one the honey, squeezed orange, lime juice, earthy-colored sugar, cinnamon, and nutmeg.

Thread the pineapple chunks onto the skewers, making a point to leave a tad of room between each piece.

Brush the pineapple skewers with the honey and zest blend, making a point to cover each piece well.

Put the skewers on the barbecue and cook for 6-8 minutes, turning every so often, until the pineapple is caramelized and lightly charred.

Eliminate the skewers from the barbecue and let them cool for a couple of moments before serving.

Discretionary: Serve the grilled pineapple skewers with a scoop of vanilla frozen yogurt or a touch of whipped cream for an additional extraordinary treat.

Partake in your tasty and healthy grilled pineapple skewers!

Integrating these salads and appetizers into your eating routine is an extraordinary method for helping your insusceptible framework and backing your general health. These dishes are loaded with fundamental supplements and nutrients that can help safeguard your body against infection and advance ideal health. Whether you're searching for a light lunch, a delectable tidbit, or an appetizer for your next gathering, these recipes make certain to please. Enjoy!

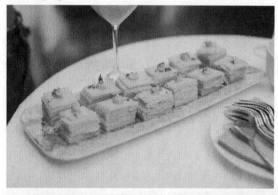

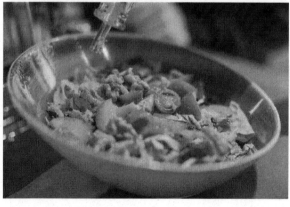

Chapter 5

Nutritious Soups and Stews to Help Fight Cancer

While there is no dependable method for forestalling cancer, a certain way of life propensities can help lessen the risk of creating it, including keeping a solid eating routine. Specifically, consuming nutritious soups and stews can be a compelling method for helping fight cancer.

Soups and stews are normally made by stewing various fixings together in a fluid base, which considers the flavors and supplements to merge. This can pursue an optimal decision for cancer patients, as they are frequently simpler to eat and process than strong food sources, and can be loaded with nutrients, minerals, and other beneficial mixtures.

Here are a few nutritious soups and stews that might help fight cancer:

Vegetable Soup

This exemplary soup is an extraordinary method for getting an assortment of cancer-fighting vegetables into your eating regimen. Vegetables like carrots, broccoli, spinach, and kale are wealthy in cell reinforcements and other beneficial mixtures that can help safeguard against cancer. Furthermore, the fluid base of the soup can help keep you hydrated, which is significant for general well-being.

Fixings
- ☐ 1 tablespoon olive oil
- ☐ 1 onion, chopped

- ☐ 2 garlic cloves, minced
- ☐ 2 carrots, chopped
- ☐ 2 celery stems, chopped
- ☐ 1 zucchini, chopped
- ☐ 1 yellow squash, chopped
- ☐ 1 can (14.5 oz) diced tomatoes
- ☐ 6 cups vegetable stock
- ☐ 1 teaspoon dried thyme
- ☐ 1 teaspoon dried oregano
- ☐ 1 teaspoon salt
- ☐ 1/2 teaspoon dark pepper
- ☐ 1 cup frozen peas
- ☐ 1 cup frozen corn
- ☐ 1 can (15 oz) chickpeas, depleted and flushed
- ☐ 2 cups new spinach, chopped
- ☐ Parmesan cheddar, ground (discretionary)

Guidelines

In an enormous pot or Dutch broiler, heat the olive oil over medium intensity.

Add the onion and garlic and cook until the onion is clear, around 5 minutes.

Add the carrots, celery, zucchini, and yellow squash to the pot and cook for an additional 5 minutes, blending at times.

Add the diced tomatoes, vegetable stock, thyme, oregano, salt, and pepper to the pot. Heat the soup to the point of boiling, then, at that point, lessen the intensity and stew for 20 minutes.

Add the frozen peas, corn, and chickpeas to the pot and cook for another 5-10 minutes, until the vegetables are delicate and the soup is warmed through.

Add the chopped spinach to the pot and mix until withered, around 1-2 minutes.

Serve the soup hot, decorated with ground Parmesan cheddar whenever wanted.

This vegetable soup recipe is an extraordinary method for spending leftover vegetables and can be effectively customized to suit your preferences. You can add different vegetables like ringer peppers, mushrooms, or yams, and change the flavors as you would prefer.

Lentil Stew

Lentils are an extraordinary wellspring of plant-based protein and fiber, which can help keep you feeling full and fulfilled. They additionally contain beneficial mixtures, for example, folate and magnesium, which have been displayed to help decrease the risk of specific cancers. Lentil stew is not difficult to make and can be enhanced with different spices and flavors for added sustenance and flavor.

Fixings
- ☐ 1 cup of dried lentils
- ☐ 1 tablespoon olive oil
- ☐ 1 huge onion, chopped

- ☐ 2 garlic cloves, minced
- ☐ 2 medium-sized carrots, chopped
- ☐ 2 stems of celery, chopped
- ☐ 1 teaspoon cumin
- ☐ 1 teaspoon paprika
- ☐ 1 teaspoon dried thyme
- ☐ 1 sound leaf
- ☐ 4 cups vegetable stock or water
- ☐ Salt and dark pepper, to taste

Chopped new parsley, for embellishing (discretionary)

Directions

Wash the lentils and put them away.

In an enormous pot or Dutch broiler, heat the olive oil over medium intensity.

Add the chopped onions and garlic and cook until the onions are clear, around 5 minutes.

Add the chopped carrots and celery and keep cooking for an additional 5 minutes or until the vegetables are delicate.

Add the cumin, paprika, and thyme, and cook for one more moment or until the flavors are fragrant.

Add the lentils, cover leaf, and vegetable stock or water to the pot and heat to the point of boiling.

Lessen the intensity to low and allow the lentils to stew for 25-30 minutes or until they are delicate.

Season with salt and dark pepper, to taste.

Decorate with chopped new parsley, whenever wanted.
Serve hot with bread or rice.

Tips
You can add more vegetables to the stew, like potatoes, yams, or tomatoes.

If you favor a thicker stew, you can mix a portion of the cooked lentils and vegetables before adding them back to the pot.

Leftover lentil stew can be stored in a sealed shut compartment in the refrigerator for up to 3-4 days or in the cooler for as long as 90 days.

Chicken Noodle Soup

While there is no conclusive proof that chicken noodle soup can fix a cold, it has for some time been utilized as a home solution for different infirmities. Chicken soup can likewise be a decent wellspring of protein and hydration, which are significant for cancer patients. Also, the carrots, celery, and different vegetables in the soup can give extra sustenance.

Fixings

- ☐ 1 pound boneless, skinless chicken bosoms
- ☐ 1 tablespoon olive oil

- ☐ 1 huge onion, chopped
- ☐ 3 carrots, stripped and chopped
- ☐ 3 celery stems, chopped
- ☐ 2 garlic cloves, minced
- ☐ 1 teaspoon dried thyme
- ☐ 1/2 teaspoon dried rosemary
- ☐ 8 cups chicken stock
- ☐ 2 cups egg noodles
- ☐ Salt and pepper to taste

New parsley, chopped (discretionary)

Guidelines

In an enormous pot or Dutch broiler, heat the olive oil over medium-high intensity.

Add the chicken bosoms and cook for 5-7 minutes on each side or until caramelized. Eliminate the chicken from the pot and put it away.

Add the onion, carrots, and celery to the pot and cook for 5-7 minutes or until the vegetables are delicate and delicate.

Add the garlic, thyme, and rosemary, and cook for an extra moment or until fragrant.

Empty the chicken stock into the pot and heat it to the point of boiling. Decrease the intensity to medium-low and let the soup stew for 10-15 minutes.

While the soup is stewing, shred the cooked chicken into little pieces utilizing two forks.

Add the egg noodles to the pot and let them cook for 7-8 minutes or until delicate.

Add the destroyed chicken back to the pot and let it heat through for 2-3 minutes.

Season the soup with salt and pepper to taste.

Serve the soup hot, decorated with chopped parsley whenever wanted.

Partake in your heavenly and encouraging chicken noodle soup!

Tomato Soup

Tomatoes are a rich wellspring of lycopene, a strong cell reinforcement that has been displayed to help safeguard against specific kinds of cancer. Tomato soup can be made with new or canned tomatoes and can be seasoned with spices and flavors for added nourishment and flavor.

Fixings

- ☐ 2 tablespoons margarine
- ☐ 1 medium onion, chopped
- ☐ 2 cloves garlic, minced
- ☐ 2 tablespoons regular baking flour
- ☐ 4 cups chicken or vegetable stock
- ☐ 2 jars (28 ounces every) of entire stripped tomatoes, undrained
- ☐ 1 teaspoon salt
- ☐ 1/4 teaspoon dark pepper
- ☐ 1/4 teaspoon sugar

☐ 1/2 cup weighty cream (discretionary)

Guidelines

In an enormous pot or Dutch broiler, dissolve the spread over medium intensity. Add the chopped onion and garlic and cook until relaxed, blending infrequently.

Sprinkle the flour over the onions and garlic and mix to join. Cook for 1-2 minutes until the flour is softly sautéed.

Pour in the chicken or vegetable stock and mix to join. Add the entire stripped tomatoes (with their juice) to the pot and mix once more.

Carry the soup to a stew and cook for 20-25 minutes, blending periodically, until the tomatoes have separated and the soup has thickened marginally.

Eliminate the soup from the intensity and permit it to cool somewhat. Utilize a submersion blender or move the soup to a blender in clumps and mix until smooth.

Return the soup to the pot and mix in the salt, dark pepper, and sugar. In the case of utilizing weighty cream, mix it in at this point.

Heat the soup over low intensity until warmed through, blending periodically. Serve hot.

Note

This recipe makes around 6-8 servings.

If you don't have a submersion blender or standard blender, you can likewise utilize a potato masher to separate the tomatoes before mixing in the salt, pepper, and sugar. You can likewise add different flavors to taste, like dried basil, oregano, or thyme.

Mushroom Soup

Mushrooms are a rich wellspring of beta-glucans, intensifies that have been displayed to help support the invulnerable framework and fight cancer. Mushroom soup can be made with various mushrooms, like shiitake, cremini, or portobello, and can be enhanced with spices and flavors for added sustenance and flavor.

Fixings

- ☐ 1 pound of new mushrooms
- ☐ 4 tablespoons of margarine
- ☐ 1 little onion, finely chopped
- ☐ 2 cloves of garlic, minced
- ☐ 4 cups of chicken or vegetable stock
- ☐ 1 cup of weighty cream
- ☐ Salt and pepper to taste
- ☐ Chopped new parsley for embellish

Guidelines

Clean the mushrooms: Eliminate any soil or trash from the mushrooms with a soggy material or paper towel. Cut the mushrooms into little pieces and put them away.

In a huge pot, soften the margarine over medium intensity. Add the finely chopped onion and minced garlic to the pot, mixing sporadically until they become delicate and fragrant.

Add the cut mushrooms to the pot, blending once in a while until they become delicate and begin to deliver their fluid. This ought to require around 5-7 minutes.

Pour the chicken or vegetable stock into the pot and heat it to the point of boiling. Lessen the intensity to low and allow it to stew for 10-15 minutes.

Eliminate the pot from the intensity and let it cool for a couple of moments. Then, utilize a submersion blender or a standard blender to puree the soup until it is smooth.

Return the soup to the pot and add the weighty cream. Heat the soup over low intensity, blending every so often, until it is warmed through.

Season the soup with salt and pepper to taste. Serve hot, decorated with chopped new parsley.

You can involve any kind of mushrooms for this recipe, however, it's ideal to utilize various mushrooms to add more profundity to the flavor.

On the off chance that you don't have a drenching blender or a customary blender, you can utilize a potato masher or a food processor to puree the soup.

You can likewise add different fixings to the soup, like thyme, rosemary, or a sprinkle of white wine, to upgrade the flavor.

Minestrone Soup

A hearty soup made with a variety of vegetables, beans, and pasta is known as a minestrone. The beans and pasta in minestrone can provide protein and fiber, and the vegetables can provide a variety of beneficial compounds. You can modify this soup to suit your preferences and nutritional requirements by adding various vegetables and herbs.

Ingredients

- ☐ 2 tablespoons olive oil
- ☐ 1 large chopped onion
- ☐ 2 minced cloves of garlic
- ☐ 2 stalks chopped celery
- ☐ 2 medium chopped carrots
- ☐ 2 medium chopped zucchini
- ☐ 1 can diced tomatoes (14.5 oz)
- ☐ 6 cups vegetable broth
- ☐ 1 can cannellini bean drained and rinsed
- ☐ 15 oz 1 cup uncooked small pasta
- ☐ 2 cups chopped kale or spinach
- ☐ 1/4 cup chopped fresh parsley Salt and pepper to taste

Directions

In a large pot, heat olive oil over medium heat.

Cook the chopped onion for about 5 minutes before adding it back in.

Cook for an additional minute before adding the minced garlic.

Cook the chopped carrots and celery for five to seven minutes, or until they begin to soften.

Cook for an additional five minutes after adding the chopped zucchini.

Stir in the diced tomatoes from the can.

Bring the soup to a simmer and add the vegetable broth.

Add the red kidney beans and cannellini beans and mix well.

Add the uncooked pasta and stew until the pasta is cooked, around 10 minutes.

Cook for another two to three minutes, or until the chopped spinach or kale wilts, before adding it.

Add the chopped parsley and stir.

To taste, add salt and pepper to the soup.

Hot, with some crusty bread on the side, serve the minestrone.
Partake in your delectable Minestrone Soup!

Stew Beef

Beef stew can provide cancer patients with important nutrients like protein, iron, and other nutrients. Potatoes, carrots, and onions, among other vegetables, can add flavor and nutrition. However, selecting lean beef cuts and limiting the stew's saturated fat content is crucial.

Ingredients

- ☐ 2 pounds of beef stew meat, cut into 1-inch cubes
- ☐ 1/4 cup all-purpose flour

- [ ] 2 tablespoons of olive oil
- [ ] 2 cups of beef broth
- [ ] 1 cup of red wine
- [ ] 1 large onion, chopped
- [ ] 4 cloves of minced garlic
- [ ] 4 medium carrots, peeled and chopped
- [ ] 3 medium potatoes, peeled and chopped
- [ ] 2 celery stalks, chopped
- [ ] 1 teaspoon dried thyme
- [ ] 1 bay leaf
- [ ] Salt and pepper to taste
- [ ] Freshly chopped parsley, for garnish
- [ ]

Directions

Turn the oven on to 350°F.

Season the beef cubes with salt and pepper in a large bowl. Toss the beef with the flour until it is evenly coated.

Olive oil should be heated to a medium-high temperature in a large Dutch oven or heavy pot. Cook the beef cubes for about 5 minutes, or until browned on all sides. Set the beef cubes aside after taking them out of the pot.

Add the hacked onion and garlic to the pot and cook until the onion is clear, around 5 minutes.

Scraping the bottom of the pot to loosen any browned bits, add the beef broth and red wine to the pot, and bring to a simmer.

Return the hamburger shapes to the pot and add the cleaved carrots, potatoes, and celery.

Add the bay leaf and dried thyme by stirring. To taste, season with salt and pepper.

Place the pot in the preheated oven and cover it with a lid. Cook the beef and vegetables for two to three hours, or until they are tender.

The bay leaf should be thrown out when you remove the pot from the oven. Season the stew according to your tastes.

Freshly chopped parsley should be added as a garnish to the hot beef stew.

It's over! Enjoy your mouth watering beef stew.

Other dietary habits can help lower the risk of developing cancer, in addition to choosing hearty stews and soups. These are some:

Consuming a variety of Vegetables and Fruits: Leafy foods contain different useful mixtures that can help safeguard against malignant growth. Expect to eat different varieties and kinds of foods grown from the ground to get the most advantage.

Whole grain options: It has been demonstrated that whole grains like brown rice, quinoa, and whole wheat bread, which are high in fiber, vitamins, and minerals, can lower the risk of certain types of cancer.

Restricting Red and Processed Meat: Red meat, such as beef and pork, should be consumed in moderation, whereas processed meats like sausage and bacon have been linked to an increased risk of cancer.

Consuming a lot of water: Remaining hydrated is significant for generally speaking well-being, and can likewise assist with diminishing the risk of specific kinds of malignant growth.

Keeping away from sweet beverages: Sweet beverages, for example, pop and natural product juice can be high in calories and can add to weight gain, which is a risk factor for some sorts of malignant growth.

Reducing Alcohol Intake: Certain types of cancer, including breast and colorectal cancer, have been linked to alcohol consumption. Be careful not to overindulge in alcoholic beverages.

To lower your risk of developing cancer, in addition to these dietary practices, it is essential to exercise regularly, maintain a healthy weight, and refrain from using tobacco products.

In conclusion, eating nutritious stews and soups can aid in the fight against cancer. These dishes are a good option for cancer patients because they can provide a variety of beneficial nutrients and are easy to digest. By integrating various nutritious food sources into your eating routine and keeping up with a sound way of life, you can assist with decreasing your risk of creating disease and advance generally speaking well-being and prosperity.

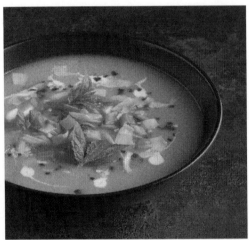

Soup

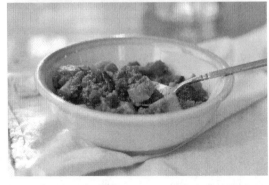

Stew

Chapter 6

Main Courses That Are Good for Your Skin

The food we devour assumes an essential part in maintaining healthy, glowing skin. Eating an even eating regimen that incorporates fundamental nutrients, minerals, and supplements can assist with forestalling skin conditions like skin inflammation, kinks, and dryness.

We will talk about a few main course standard healthy meals that are great for your skin. These meals are nutritious as well as delectable, and they will leave you feeling fulfilled and nourished.

Grilled Salmon with Quinoa and Roasted Vegetables

Salmon is an incredible wellspring of omega-3 unsaturated fats, which are fundamental for maintaining healthy skin. Omega-3 unsaturated fats help to lessen aggravation, which can cause skin conditions like skin breakout and psoriasis. Quinoa is a gluten grain that is high in protein and fiber, making it a great wellspring of sustenance for the body. Roasted vegetables like sweet potatoes, carrots, and broccoli are plentiful in nutrients A, C, and E, which are fundamental for healthy skin.

To make this dish, begin by preparing the salmon with salt, pepper, and lemon juice. Barbecue the salmon for 5-7 minutes on each side until it is cooked through. While the salmon is cooking, set up the quinoa by bubbling 1 cup of quinoa in 2 cups of water. Once the quinoa is cooked, cushion it with a fork and put it away. Cut the vegetables into scaled-down pieces and meal them in the broiler for 20-25 minutes until they are delicate.

To serve, put a serving of quinoa on the plate, top it with the grilled salmon, and serve the roasted vegetables as an afterthought.

Turkey Bean stew with Brown Rice

Turkey is an extraordinary wellspring of lean protein, which is fundamental for building and fixing skin tissue. It is likewise low in fat, making it a better choice than meat. Stew is an extraordinary method for integrating various vegetables into your eating regimen, which are plentiful in nutrients and minerals that are fundamental for healthy skin. Brown rice is a complicated starch that is high in fiber, making it a phenomenal wellspring of energy for the body.

To make this dish, begin by browning 1 pound of ground turkey in a huge pot. When the turkey is cooked, add diced onions, chime peppers, and garlic to the pot and cook until the vegetables are delicate. Add diced tomatoes, kidney beans, stew powder, cumin, and paprika to the pot, and stew for 20-30 minutes until the flavors have merged.

While the bean stew is cooking, set up the brown rice by bubbling 1 cup of rice in 2 cups of water. When the rice is cooked, cushion it with a fork and put it away.

To serve, put a serving of brown rice on the plate, top it with a serving of bean stew, and trim with chopped cilantro.

Grilled Chicken with Sweet Potato Pound and Steamed Green Beans

Chicken is an incredible wellspring of lean protein, which is fundamental for building and fixing skin tissue. Sweet potatoes are plentiful in beta-carotene, which is changed over into vitamin A in the body. Vitamin A is fundamental for healthy skin, as it assists with directing the creation of sebum, which can cause skin break out. Green beans are plentiful in L-ascorbic acid, which is fundamental for collagen creation in the skin.

To make this dish, begin by preparing the chicken with salt, pepper, and your number one spices. Barbecue the chicken for 5-7 minutes on each side until it is cooked through. While the chicken is cooking, strip, and hack 2 sweet potatoes into little pieces. Heat the sweet potatoes in a pot of water until they are delicate, then, at that point, crush them with a fork or potato masher. Add a sprinkle of milk and spread for additional smoothness whenever wanted.

To steam the green beans, place them in a liner bin and steam for 3-4 minutes until they are delicate yet fresh.

To serve, place a serving of sweet potato pound on the plate, top it with the grilled chicken, and serve the steamed green beans as an afterthought.

Lentil and Vegetable Sautéed food with Brown Rice

Lentils are a superb wellspring of plant-based protein and fiber, making them an incredible expansion to any eating routine. They are additionally wealthy in iron, which is fundamental for healthy skin. Vegetables, for example, ringer peppers, carrots, and broccoli are plentiful in nutrients A, C, and E, which are fundamental for healthy skin.

To make this dish, begin by cooking 1 cup of brown rice in 2 cups of water. When the rice is cooked, cushion it with a fork and put it away. In a huge skillet, heat some oil and add diced onions and garlic. When the onions are clear, add diced chime peppers, carrots, and broccoli to the dish and sautéed food for 3-4 minutes until the vegetables are delicate yet at the same time fresh. Add 1 cup of cooked lentils to the dish and pan-fried food for an extra 2-3 minutes until the lentils are warmed through.

To serve, put a serving of brown rice on the plate, top it with a serving of lentil and vegetable pan-fried food, and enhance with cleaved cilantro.

Baked Cod with Roasted Vegetables and Quinoa Salad

Cod is an extraordinary wellspring of lean protein, which is fundamental for building and fixing skin tissue. It is likewise plentiful in vitamin D, which is fundamental for healthy skin. Roasted vegetables like sweet potatoes, carrots, and Brussels sprouts are plentiful in nutrients A, C, and E, which are fundamental for healthy skin. Quinoa salad is an extraordinary method for integrating different vegetables into your eating routine, which are plentiful in nutrients and minerals that are fundamental for healthy skin.

To make this dish, begin by preparing the cod with salt, pepper, and lemon juice. Prepare the cod on the stove for 15-20 minutes until it is cooked through. While the cod is heating up, cut the vegetables into scaled-down pieces and dish them in the broiler for 20-25 minutes until they are delicate.

To make the quinoa salad, cook 1 cup of quinoa in 2 cups of water. Once the quinoa is cooked, cushion it with a fork and put it away. In an enormous bowl, combine one diced cucumber, tomatoes, red onion, and chime peppers. Add the cooked quinoa to the bowl and blend until everything is very much consolidated. Sprinkle with olive oil and lemon juice for additional character.

To serve, put a serving of quinoa salad on the plate, top it with the baked cod, and serve the roasted vegetables as an afterthought.

Spinach and Feta Stuffed Chicken Bosom

Fixings
- ☐ 4 boneless, skinless chicken bosoms
- ☐ 2 cups of new spinach leaves
- ☐ 1/2 cup disintegrated feta cheddar
- ☐ 2 cloves garlic, minced
- ☐ 1 tablespoon olive oil
- ☐ Salt and pepper, to taste
- ☐ Toothpicks or kitchen twine (discretionary)

Directions
Preheat your stove to 375°F (190°C).

Wash the chicken bosoms and wipe them off with paper towels.

Cut a pocket into every chicken bosom by cutting on a level plane into the thickest piece of the bosom, being mindful so as not to carve the entire way through. The pocket ought to be adequately huge to stuff the filling inside.

In a skillet over medium intensity, sauté the minced garlic in the olive oil until fragrant, around 30 seconds.

Add the spinach onto the skillet and cook until shriveled, around 2-3 minutes.

Eliminate the skillet from the intensity and mix in the disintegrated feta cheddar. Blend well to join.

Utilize a spoon to stuff the spinach and feta combination into the pockets of the chicken bosoms. Use toothpicks or kitchen twine to get the opening and keep the filling inside (discretionary).

Season the chicken bosoms with salt and pepper, to taste.

Heat a skillet over medium-high intensity and add a tablespoon of olive oil.

Add the stuffed chicken bosoms to the skillet and cook for around 2-3 minutes on each side or until brilliant brown.

Move the skillet to the preheated stove and prepare for 20-25 minutes, or until the chicken is cooked through and presently not pink in the center.

Eliminate the toothpicks or kitchen twine from the chicken bosoms and let them rest for 5 minutes before serving.

Serve the Spinach and Feta stuffed chicken bosom hot, decorated with new spices, whenever wanted. Enjoy!

Eating healthy meals that are plentiful in nutrients, minerals, and supplements is fundamental for maintaining healthy, glowing skin. Consolidating different lean proteins, entire grains, and vegetables into your eating routine can assist with forestalling skin conditions like skin break out, kinks, and dryness. By observing these main course guidelines for healthy meals, you can sustain your body and your skin, leaving you feeling fulfilled and great.

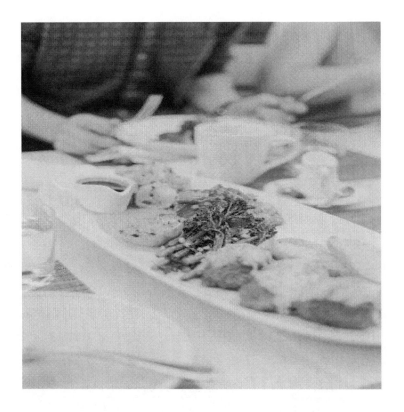

Chapter 7

Healthy Snacks and Desserts for Skin Protection

A balanced diet with fundamental supplements assists with keeping our skin healthy and gleaming. Nonetheless, sometimes we will more often than not enjoy unhealthy snacking, which can antagonistically affect our skin. To guarantee that we keep up with healthy skin, we should consume healthy snacks and desserts that advance skin protection.

We will discuss the significance of healthy snacks and desserts for skin protection, some healthy bite and dessert choices, and how they benefit our skin.

Significance of Healthy Snacks and Desserts for Skin Protection:

The skin is the biggest organ in the human body and goes about as a defensive hindrance against outer components. The skin's well-being is straightforwardly connected with our general well-being, and unfortunate nutrition can prompt different skin issues like skin inflammation, wrinkles, dry skin, and dark circles. Polishing off unhealthy snacks and desserts like chips, sweet beverages, and chocolates can prompt a lopsidedness in the body, bringing about irritation, which can prompt skin issues.

Therefore, it is fundamental to consume healthy snacks and desserts that are plentiful in vitamins, minerals, and cancer prevention agents to advance skin protection. These snacks and desserts can assist with lessening irritation, preventing skin break out, dialing back the maturing system, and keeping the skin hydrated and sparkling.

Healthy Snack Choices for Skin Protection

Nuts and Seeds
Nuts and seeds are a rich source of fundamental unsaturated fats, minerals, and vitamins that are urgent for healthy skin. They contain omega-3 and omega-6 unsaturated fats that assist to lessen aggravation, which can cause skin inflammation and other skin issues. Some instances of nuts and seeds that are perfect for snacking incorporate almonds, pecans, pumpkin seeds, and sunflower seeds.

Fruits
Fruits are a superb source of vitamins, minerals, and cell reinforcements that advance healthy skin. They contain vitamin C, which assists with helping collagen

production, and keeps the skin firm and flexible. Fruits like berries, kiwis, mangoes, and oranges are wealthy in cell reinforcements that assist to shield the skin from harm brought about by free revolutionaries.

Vegetables

Vegetables are an incredible source of vitamins, minerals, and cell reinforcements that are fundamental for healthy skin. They contain vitamin A, which assists with preventing skin inflammation and kinks, and vitamin C, which assists with helping collagen production. Vegetables like carrots, yams, broccoli, and spinach are perfect for snacking and give various benefits to the skin.

Greek Yogurt

Greek yogurt is an extraordinary source of protein, which assists with advancing healthy skin. It contains probiotics, which can assist with diminishing aggravation and prevent skin break out. Greek yogurt is also wealthy in calcium, which assists with keeping the skin firm and healthy.

Healthy Dessert Choices for Skin Protection

Dark Chocolate

Dark chocolate is a rich source of cell reinforcements that assist to safeguard the skin from harm brought about by free revolutionaries. It also contains flavonoids, which can assist with decreasing irritation and further develop a bloodstream to the skin. Dark chocolate with a high level of cocoa is the most ideal choice for advancing skin protection.

Berries and Cream

Berries like strawberries, blueberries, and raspberries are an incredible source of cell reinforcements that advance healthy skin. Adding whipped cream produced using Greek yogurt to berries makes for a flavorful and healthy dessert choice that gives various skin benefits.

Chia Seed Pudding

Chia seeds are a rich source of omega-3 unsaturated fats, which help to diminish irritation and advance healthy skin. Chia seed pudding made with almond milk, honey, and fruit is a scrumptious and healthy dessert choice that gives various skin benefits.

Avocado Chocolate Mousse

Avocado is an extraordinary source of healthy fats, vitamins, and minerals that are fundamental for healthy skin. Avocado chocolate mousse is a tasty and healthy dessert choice that gives various skin benefits. Avocado is plentiful in vitamin E, which assists with shielding the skin from harm brought about by free revolutionaries. It also contains healthy fats that assist to keep the skin hydrated and prevent wrinkles.

How Healthy Snacks and Desserts Benefit Skin

Reduces Aggravation

Irritation is one of the main sources of skin issues like skin inflammation, kinks, and dry skin. Consuming healthy snacks and desserts that are wealthy in cell reinforcements, omega-3 unsaturated fats, and probiotics can assist with diminishing irritation and advance healthy skin.

Advances Collagen Production

Collagen is a protein that is fundamental for healthy skin. It assists with keeping the skin firm and graceful. Consuming snacks and desserts that are plentiful in vitamin C, like fruits and vegetables, can assist with advancing collagen production, which can dial back the maturing system and keep the skin looking young.

Keeps the Skin Hydrated

Consuming healthy snacks and desserts that are wealthy in healthy fats, like nuts, seeds, and avocado, can assist with keeping the skin hydrated. Hydrated skin is less inclined to kinks and dryness, which can prompt skin issues.

Shields the Skin from Harm

Healthy snacks and desserts that are wealthy in cell reinforcements, like dark chocolate and berries, can assist with shielding the skin from harm brought about by free extremists. Free revolutionaries are unsteady particles that can harm the skin and cause untimely maturing.

Cautiously note; consuming healthy snacks and desserts is fundamental for advancing skin protection. They give fundamental supplements that are pivotal for healthy skin, like vitamins, minerals, cell reinforcements, and omega-3 unsaturated fats. Healthy snacks and desserts can assist with diminishing irritation, advance collagen production, keep the skin hydrated, and safeguard the skin from harm brought about by free revolutionaries.

While picking healthy snacks and desserts for skin protection, it is fundamental to settle on choices that are wealthy in fundamental supplements and low in sugar and unhealthy fats. Integrating these healthy snacks and desserts into your everyday diet can assist with advancing healthy skin and preventing skin cancer.

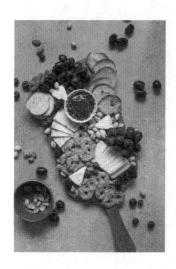

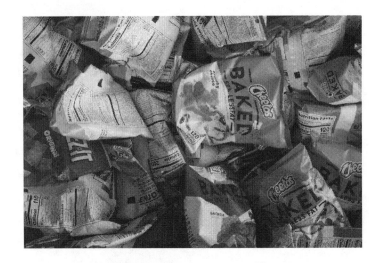

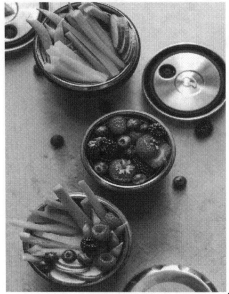

Desserts

Chapter 8

<u>Beverages that Help Prevent Skin Cancer</u>

Beverages that help prevent skin cancer are important for all types of people beyond 40 years old. Skin cancer is a typical type of cancer, and it is caused by openness to the sun's ultraviolet (UV) rays. While it is important to protect your skin with sunscreen and protective clothing, certain beverages can also help to prevent skin cancer by furnishing your body with important nutrients and antioxidants that protect against damage from UV rays.

One of the most important beverages for preventing skin cancer is green tea. Green tea is wealthy in antioxidants called catechins, which help to protect the skin against damage from UV rays. Catechins also have anti-inflammatory properties, which can help to decrease the risk of skin cancer by diminishing inflammation in the skin. Studies have demonstrated the way that drinking green tea can help to lessen the risk of creating skin cancer, particularly squamous cell carcinoma, which is the second most normal type of skin cancer.

Another beverage that can help to prevent skin cancer is red wine. Red wine contains resveratrol, a strong antioxidant that has been displayed to protect the skin against damage from UV rays. Resveratrol also has anti-inflammatory properties, which can help to diminish the risk of skin cancer by lessening inflammation in the skin.

Studies have shown that drinking moderate amounts of red wine can help to decrease the risk of creating skin cancer, particularly basal cell carcinoma, which is the most widely recognized type of skin cancer.

In addition to green tea and red wine, other beverages that can help to prevent skin cancer include:

Water: Staying hydrated is important for maintaining healthy skin. Drinking plenty of water can help to keep your skin hydrated and prevent dryness, which can make your skin more susceptible to damage from UV rays.

Coconut water: Coconut water is wealthy in potassium, which helps to keep your skin hydrated and prevent dryness. It also contains antioxidants that protect against damage from UV rays.

Tomato Juice: Tomatoes are wealthy in lycopene, a strong antioxidant that helps to protect the skin against damage from UV rays. Drinking tomato juice can help to give your body lycopene and other important nutrients that protect against skin cancer.

Carrot Juice: Carrots are wealthy in beta-carotene, a nutrient that helps to protect the skin against damage from UV rays. Drinking carrot juice can help to give your body beta-carotene and other important nutrients that protect against skin cancer.

Pomegranate Juice: Pomegranate juice is wealthy in antioxidants, including polyphenols, which help to protect the skin against damage from UV rays. Drinking pomegranate juice can help to give your body these important antioxidants and decrease the risk of skin cancer.

Kombucha - a fermented tea that is a great wellspring of probiotics and antioxidants.

Chai Tea - a flavored tea that is often delighted in with milk and honey.

Bone Broth - a nutrient-rich broth made from stewing bones and connective tissue.

Sparkling water with a splash of fruit juice - an invigorating and low-calorie alternative to soda.

Matcha green Tea - is a powdered tea that is high in antioxidants and caffeine.

Herbal Tea - a non-caffeinated tea that can be delightful in hot or cold and offers a variety of health benefits.

Soda - a carbonated beverage with ginger, which can help with digestion and nausea.

Non-alcoholic lager or wine - a great option for those who want the taste of brew or wine without the alcohol.

It is important to note that while these beverages can help to prevent skin cancer, they ought not to be utilized as a substitute for sunscreen and protective clothing. It is still important to protect your skin from UV rays by wearing protective clothing and applying sunscreen with an SPF of 30 or higher. In addition, it is important to limit your openness to the sun, particularly during peak hours when the sun's rays are the strongest.

All in all, incorporating beverages that help to prevent skin cancer into your daily routine is a straightforward and effective way to protect your skin against damage from UV rays. Green tea, red wine, water, coconut water, tomato juice, carrot juice, and pomegranate juice are all excellent options that give your body important nutrients and antioxidants that protect against skin cancer. In any case, it is important to recollect that these beverages ought to be utilized in conjunction with other sun protection methods, like wearing protective clothing and applying sunscreen. By taking these steps, you can help to lessen your risk of creating skin cancer and maintain healthy, beautiful skin.

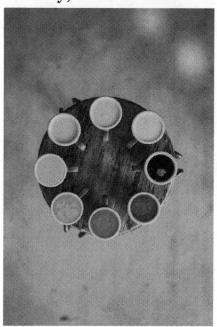

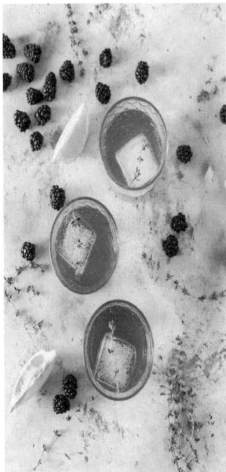

Beverages

Chapter 9

Meal Plan

Weekly Meal Plan with Recipes

Skin cancer is one of the most widely recognized types of cancer, and the risk of creating it increments as we age. A sound diet can assist with decreasing the risk of creating skin cancer, and integrating specific food varieties can help safeguard against it. This weekly meal plan is intended to give men and women beyond 40 years old a solid and tasty Anti-Skin Cancer Diet.

Morning

Breakfast is much of the time called the main meal of the day and for good explanation. It establishes the vibe until the end of the day and furnishes the body with the fuel it necessities to appropriately work. For a skin cancer diet, it's essential to pick food varieties that are plentiful in cell reinforcements, nutrients, and minerals.

Monday

Smoothie Bowl: Mix 1 cup of frozen blended berries, 1 banana, 1/2 cup of unsweetened almond milk, 1 tablespoon of chia seeds, and 1 tablespoon of honey until smooth. Empty the blend into a bowl and top with 1/4 cup of granola and a modest bunch of new blueberries.

Tuesday

Avocado Toast: Toast 2 cuts of entire grain bread and spread 1/2 an avocado on each cut.

Top with cut cherry tomatoes, a sprinkle of ocean salt, and a shower of olive oil.

Wednesday

Greek Yogurt Parfait: In a container or bowl, layer 1 cup of plain Greek yogurt, 1/2 cup of blended berries, 1 tablespoon of honey, and 1/4 cup of granola.

Thursday

Veggie Omelet: Beat 2 eggs with a sprinkle of almond milk. Heat a non-stick skillet over medium-high intensity and add 1/2 cup of cut mushrooms, 1/2 cup of hacked spinach, and 1/4 cup of diced tomatoes. Pour the egg blend over the veggies and cook until set. Overlay the omelet down the middle and serve.

Friday

Peanut Margarine and Banana Toast: Toast 2 cuts of entire grain bread and spread 2 tablespoons of normal peanut margarine on each cut. Top with a cut banana and a sprinkle of cinnamon.

Saturday

Blueberry Flapjacks: In a bowl, blend 1 cup of entire wheat flour, 2 teaspoons of baking powder, 1/2 teaspoon of cinnamon, and a touch of salt. In a different bowl, whisk together 1 egg, 1/2 cup of unsweetened almond milk, 1 tablespoon of honey, and 1/2 teaspoon of vanilla concentrate. Empty the wet fixings into the dry fixings and mix until recently consolidated. Overlay in 1 cup of new blueberries. Heat a non-stick skillet over medium intensity and spoon 1/4 cup of player for every hotcake. Cook until the edges begin to dry and the air pockets in the middle pop. Flip the flapjack and cook for one more moment or until brilliant brown.

Sunday

Breakfast Burrito: Intensity a non-stick skillet over medium-high intensity and add 1/2 cup of cut mushrooms, 1/4 cup of diced onion, and 1/4 cup of diced chime pepper. Cook until the veggies are delicate. In a different bowl, whisk together 2 eggs and 1 tablespoon of unsweetened almond milk. Add the egg combination to the skillet and cook until set. Spoon the egg combination onto an entire grain tortilla and top with 1/4 cup of destroyed cheddar cheese and a bit of salsa. Roll the tortilla and serve.

Afternoon

Lunch is a significant meal that gives the body the energy it necessities to get past the day. For an Anti of a skin cancer diet, it's essential to pick food sources that are plentiful in nutrients, and minerals.

Monday

Barbecued Chicken Serving of mixed greens: Barbecue 4 ounces of chicken bosom and cut it into strips. In a bowl, blend 2 cups of leafy greens, 1/4 cup of cut cucumber, 1/4 cup of cherry tomatoes, and 1/4 cup of cut avocado. Top with the chicken fingers and sprinkle with a combination of 1 tablespoon of olive oil and 1 tablespoon of balsamic vinegar.

Tuesday

Quinoa and Dark Bean Bowl: In a bowl, blend 1 cup of cooked quinoa, 1/2 cup of dark beans, 1/4 cup of diced red onion, 1/4 cup of diced ringer pepper, and 1/4 cup of corn bits. Sprinkle with a combination of 1 tablespoon of olive oil and 1 tablespoon of lime juice.

Wednesday

<u>Fish Salad Lettuce Wraps:</u> Channel a container of fish and blend it in with 1 tablespoon of mayonnaise, 1 tablespoon of diced celery, and 1 tablespoon of diced red onion. Spoon the fish salad onto 4 enormous lettuce leaves and roll them up.

<u>Thursday</u>

<u>Veggie Wrap:</u> Spread 2 tablespoons of hummus on an entire-grain tortilla. Add 1/4 cup of cut cucumber, 1/4 cup of cut chime pepper, 1/4 cup of cut carrots, and a small bunch of leafy greens. Roll the tortilla and serve.

<u>Friday</u>

<u>Turkey and Cheese Sandwich:</u> Toast 2 cuts of entire grain bread and add 2 ounces of cut turkey bosom and 1 cut of Swiss cheese. Top with cut tomato and blended greens.

Saturday

Egg Salad Sandwich: Hardly bubble 2 eggs and crush them with 1 tablespoon of mayonnaise, 1 tablespoon of diced celery, and 1 tablespoon of diced red onion. Spread the egg salad on 2 cuts of entire-grain bread and top with blended greens.

Sunday

Barbecued Veggie Panini: Intensity a panini press. Spread 2 cuts of entire grain bread with 2 tablespoons of pesto. Add 1/4 cup of cut eggplant, 1/4 cup of cut zucchini, 1/4 cup of cut ringer pepper, and 1 cup of mozzarella cheese. Barbecue the panini until the bread is toasted and the cheese is liquefied.

Evening

Dinner is the last meal of the day and ought to be offset with various supplements to advance general health. For an anti-skin cancer diet, it's critical to pick food varieties that are wealthy in antioxidants and mitigating compounds.

Monday

Grilled Salmon: Season a 4-ounce salmon filet with salt and pepper. Barbecue the salmon for 3-4 minutes for each side. Present with a side of grilled asparagus and quinoa.

Tuesday

Chicken Pan fried food: In a wok or enormous skillet, heat 1 tablespoon of sesame oil over high intensity. Add 4 ounces of cut chicken bosom and cook until seared. Eliminate the chicken from the dish and put it away. Add 1 cup of cut blended veggies, (for example, ringer pepper, onion, and carrot) to the container and cook until delicate. Add the chicken back to the dish and mix in a combination of 1 tablespoon of soy sauce and 1 tablespoon of honey. Serve over earthy-colored rice.

Wednesday

Dark Bean and Yam Tacos: In a skillet, heat 1 tablespoon of olive oil over medium intensity. Add 1 cup of diced yam and cook until delicate. Add 1/2 cup of dark beans and 1/4 cup of diced onion to the skillet and cook until warmed through. Warm 4 corn tortillas in the microwave. Split the yam and dark bean blend between the tortillas and top with diced avocado and salsa.

Thursday

Grilled Chicken Kabobs: Cut 4 ounces of chicken bosom into cubes. String the chicken onto sticks alongside 1 cup of blended veggies, (for example, ringer pepper, onion, and zucchini). Barbecue the kabobs until the chicken is cooked through. Present with a side of quinoa.

Friday

Lentil Soup: In an enormous pot, heat 1 tablespoon of olive oil over medium intensity. Add 1/2 cup of diced onion, 1/2 cup of diced carrot, and 1/2 cup of diced celery. Cook until the vegetables are delicate. Add 2 cups of low-sodium chicken stock, 1 cup of lentils, and 1 cove leaf. Heat the soup to the point of boiling, then decrease the intensity and stew for 20-25 minutes, or until the lentils are cooked through. Eliminate the cove leaf and season with salt and pepper to taste.

Saturday

Grilled Shrimp Sticks: String 8-10 huge shrimp onto sticks. Brush the shrimp with a combination of 1 tablespoon of olive oil and 1 tablespoon of lemon juice. Barbecue the sticks until the shrimp are pink and cooked through. Present with a side of grilled vegetables, (for example, zucchini, chime pepper, and onion).

Sunday

Baked Chicken Thighs: Preheat the stove or oven to 375°F. Season 2 chicken thighs with salt, pepper, and a sprinkle of paprika. Prepare the chicken for 30-35 minutes, or until cooked through. Present with a side of broiled yams or preferably sweet potatoes and steamed broccoli.

Snacks

Snacks can be a significant piece of a healthy diet, giving energy and supplements between meals. For an Anti-Skin cancer diet, it's critical to pick snacks that are wealthy in antioxidants and calming compounds.

Carrot Sticks and Hummus: Cut 1/2 cup of carrot sticks and present with 2 tablespoons of hummus.

Greek Yogurt with Berries: Blend 1/2 cup of plain Greek yogurt with a modest bunch of blended berries.

Apple Cuts with Almond Spread: Cut 1 medium apple and present with 1 tablespoon of almond margarine.

Trail Blend: Combine as one 1/4 cup of nuts, 1/4 cup of dried natural product, and 1/4 cup of entire grain oat.

Hard-Bubbled Egg: Bubble 1 egg and present with a sprinkle of salt and pepper.

Following a skin cancer diet doesn't need to be troublesome or boring. By integrating various beautiful fruits and vegetables, lean proteins, and healthy fats, you can make heavenly and fulfilling meals that help general health and lessen your risk of skin cancer. This week-after-week meal plan gives a format to a reasonable and thick diet that can assist with safeguarding your skin and advancing ideal health.

Grocery List

Keeping a healthy diet is fundamental for forestalling and lessening the risk of skin cancer. Certain food varieties contain antioxidants, nutrients, and minerals that can shield the skin from destructive UV beams and forestall skin harm. We will make a healthy and checked grocery list for people over 40 to assist with forestalling skin cancer.

Fruits and Vegetables:

Fruits and vegetables are a phenomenal wellspring of antioxidants that assist with safeguarding the skin from UV harm. They additionally contain nutrients and minerals that keep the skin healthy and energetic. The accompanying fruits and vegetables ought to be remembered for your grocery list:

Berries - Strawberries, blueberries, raspberries, and blackberries are wealthy in antioxidants that assist with shielding the skin from sun harm.

Salad greens - Kale, spinach, and other mixed greens contain elevated degrees of nutrients A, C, and E, which are significant for skin health.

Carrots - Carrots are plentiful in beta-carotene, which is changed over into vitamin A in the body. Vitamin A is fundamental for keeping up with healthy skin.

Tomatoes - Tomatoes contain lycopene, a cancer-prevention agent that safeguards the skin from UV harm.

Yams - Yams are a decent wellspring of vitamin A, which is fundamental for skin health.

Citrus fruits - Citrus fruits like oranges, lemons, and grapefruits are plentiful in L-ascorbic acid, which safeguards the skin from sun harm.

Protein - Protein is fundamental for keeping up with healthy skin. It helps fix and recover skin cells and tissues. The accompanying protein sources ought to be remembered for your grocery list:

Salmon - Salmon is an amazing wellspring of omega-3 unsaturated fats, which assist with decreasing aggravation and safeguarding the skin from UV harm.

Chicken - Chicken is a decent wellspring of protein, which is fundamental for keeping up with healthy skin.

Nuts - Nuts like almonds, walnuts, and cashews are a decent wellspring of protein and vitamin E, which shields the skin from sun harm.

Beans - Beans are a decent wellspring of protein and antioxidants that assist with shielding the skin from UV harm.

Greek Yogurt - Greek yogurt is a phenomenal wellspring of protein and probiotics, which assist with keeping up with healthy skin.

Healthy Fats

Healthy fats are fundamental for keeping up with healthy skin. They assist with keeping the skin saturated and forestall dryness and kinks. The accompanying healthy fats ought to be remembered for your grocery list:

Avocado - Avocado is a fantastic wellspring of healthy fats that assist with keeping the skin saturated and forestalling wrinkles.

Olive oil - Olive oil is wealthy in antioxidants and healthy fats that assist with safeguarding the skin from UV harm.

Flaxseeds - Flaxseeds are a decent wellspring of omega-3 unsaturated fats, which assist with diminishing irritation and safeguarding the skin from UV harm.

Coconut oil - Coconut oil is a decent wellspring of healthy fats that assist with keeping the skin saturated and forestalling wrinkles.

Drinks

Drinks likewise assume a significant part in keeping up with healthy skin. The accompanying drinks ought to be remembered for your grocery list:

Green tea - Green tea is wealthy in antioxidants that assist with shielding the skin from sun harm.

Water - Drinking a lot of water helps keep the skin hydrated and forestall dryness and kinks.

New squeeze - Newly pressed juice is an amazing wellspring of nutrients and minerals that are fundamental for skin health.

Milk - Milk is a decent wellspring of vitamin D, which is significant for keeping up with healthy skin.

Different food varieties:

Notwithstanding the previously mentioned food varieties, the accompanying food sources ought to likewise be remembered for your grocery list:

Entire grains - Entire grains like earthy colored rice, entire wheat bread, and quinoa are a decent wellspring of fiber, which keeps up with healthy skin.

Dark Chocolate - Dark chocolate contains flavonoids, which assist with safeguarding the skin from UV harm.

Garlic - Garlic contains allicin, which has calming properties and shields the skin from sun harm.

Turmeric - Turmeric contains curcumin, which has calming properties and shields the skin from sun harm.

Mushrooms - Mushrooms are a decent wellspring of vitamin D, which is significant for keeping up with healthy skin.

Red grapes - Red grapes contain resveratrol, which has mitigating properties and safeguards the skin from UV harm.

It is critical to take note that a healthy diet alone can't forestall skin cancer. Different measures, for example, wearing defensive apparel and utilizing sunscreen ought to likewise be taken to diminish the risk of skin cancer.

The previously mentioned grocery list incorporates food sources that are plentiful in antioxidants, nutrients, and minerals that are fundamental for keeping up with healthy skin and diminishing the risk of skin cancer. Integrating these food varieties into your diet can assist with safeguarding your skin from UV harm and keep it looking young and healthy.

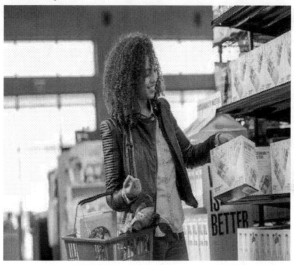

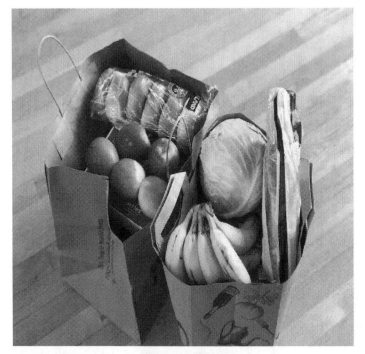

Grocery items

Chapter 10

<u>Skin Care Tips to Prevent Melanoma</u>

From the starting point of this book, we came to comprehend thatMelanoma is a sort of skin cancer that creates melanocyte cells, which produce color in the skin. While it is more uncommon than different sorts of skin cancer, it is more perilous and can be deadly whenever left untreated. Fortunately, various skin care tips can assist with preventing melanoma in people beyond 40 years old. We will investigate the best techniques for decreasing the risk of melanoma.

Use Sunscreen

Quite possibly the main step you can take to prevent melanoma is to utilize sunscreen. Sunscreen assists with shielding your skin from the destructive UV beams of the sun, which can harm the DNA in your skin cells and increment your risk of creating melanoma. While picking a sunscreen, search for one that has a high SPF (no less than 30) and gives expansive range insurance against both UVA and UVB beams.

Apply sunscreen generously to all uncovered areas of skin, including your face, neck, hands, and arms. Make certain to reapply it like clockwork or in the wake of swimming or perspiring. It is additionally critical to utilize sunscreen even on overcast days, as UV beams can in any case enter mists and cause skin harm.

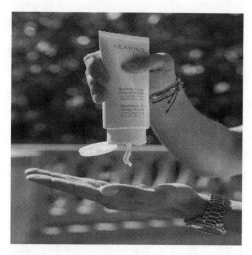

<u>Wear Defensive Attire</u>

Notwithstanding sunscreen, wearing defensive attire is one more powerful method for preventing melanoma. Clothing that covers your skin can assist with safeguarding it from the sun's destructive beams. Search for dresses produced using firmly woven textures, as these give preferable security over free, lightweight textures.

Think about wearing a wide-overflowed cap to safeguard your face and neck, and shades to shield your eyes from UV beams. On the off chance that you intend to invest a ton of energy outside, think about wearing long-sleeved shirts and jeans to cover however much of your skin as could be expected.

Try not to Tan Beds

Tanning beds discharge UV radiation, which can expand your risk of creating melanoma. Utilizing a tanning bed just once can build your risk of melanoma by 20%.

If you need a tan, think about utilizing a self-tanning moisturizer or splash all things being equal.

Perform Skin Checks

Performing normal skin checks is a significant piece of preventing melanoma. Check your skin consistently for any new moles, spots, or other uncommon developments. If you notice any progressions in your skin, like changes in variety, size, or shape, or on the other hand if a mole or spot begins to tingle, drain, or cover over, consider a dermatologist as soon as could be expected.

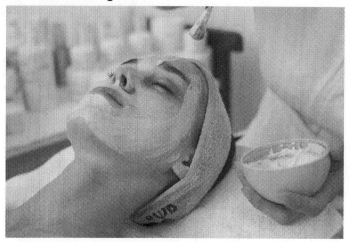

<u>Know about Your risk Variables</u>

Certain elements can expand your risk of creating melanoma, including:

- Light complexion
- Family background of melanoma
- History of sun-related burns
- Numerous moles or surprising moles
- Debilitated insusceptible framework
- Openness to UV radiation

For example, from tanning beds or sun-related burns.Assuming you have any of these risk factors, it is particularly critical to do whatever it may take to prevent melanoma.

Eat a Solid Diet

Eating a solid diet can likewise assist with decreasing your risk of melanoma. Food varieties that are wealthy in antioxidants, like products of the soil, can assist with safeguarding your skin from the harmful impacts of UV radiation. Furthermore, food varieties that are high in omega-3 unsaturated fats, like salmon and other greasy fish, can assist with lessening aggravation in your skin and safeguarding against skin harm.

Remain Hydrated

Drinking a lot of water is likewise significant for solid skin. At the point when you are dried out, your skin can become dry and more helpless to harm from the sun's beams. Mean to drink something like eight glasses of water a day to keep your skin hydrated and solid.

Stop Smoking

Smoking can expand your risk of creating melanoma, as well as different sorts of cancer. It can likewise harm your skin, making it more defenseless to UV radiation. Assuming you smoke, stopping is quite possibly the smartest option for your general well-being and the soundness of your skin.

Oversee Pressure

Ongoing pressure can debilitate your resistant framework and increase aggravation in your body, which can expand your risk of creating melanoma. Tracking down ways of overseeing pressure, like through exercise, contemplation, or investing energy in nature, can assist with decreasing your risk.

Get Normal Skin Tests

At long last, getting ordinary skin tests from a dermatologist is significant. A dermatologist can take a look at your skin for any indications of melanoma and give direction on the best way to diminish your risk. If you have a background marked by melanoma or other risk factors, your dermatologist might suggest more continuous skin tests.

Preventing melanoma requires a mix of techniques, including utilizing sunscreen and wearing a defensive dress, abstaining from tanning beds, performing customary skin checks, monitoring your risk factors, eating a solid diet, remaining hydrated, stopping smoking, overseeing pressure, and getting normal skin tests. By making these strides, you can assist with safeguarding your skin and diminish your risk of creating melanoma.

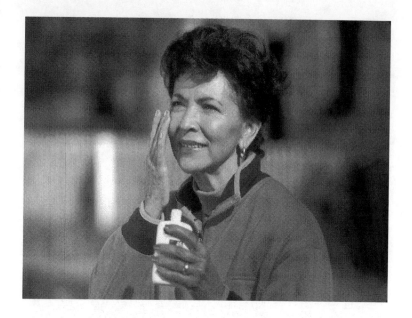

A woman in a pink jacket applies sunscreen to her face outside

<u>Conclusion</u>

As the author of this anti-skin cancer cookbook, I would like to take this opportunity to deeply emphasize the importance of supporting a healthy lifestyle in reducing the risk of skin cancer. While many people often focus on protecting their skin from harmful UV rays, they forget that a healthy lifestyle plays a vital role in preventing skin cancer.

One of the best ways to reduce the risk of skin cancer is by adopting a healthy lifestyle. This includes eating a balanced diet, exercising regularly, and avoiding harmful habits such as smoking and excessive alcohol consumption. By doing so, we can boost our immune system, which helps in fighting cancer-causing agents and reducing inflammation that could lead to skin cancer.

Eating a healthy and balanced diet is particularly essential in the prevention of skin cancer. A diet rich in fruits, vegetables, whole grains, lean proteins, and healthy fats can provide our bodies with essential nutrients that help in preventing skin cancer. For instance, foods rich in antioxidants, such as blueberries, spinach, and carrots, can protect our skin from damage caused by UV radiation.

Moreover, the power of food in fighting skin cancer cannot be underestimated. Some foods have been shown to have anti-cancer properties and can help in preventing skin cancer. For instance, studies have shown that green tea contains compounds that can help prevent skin cancer by blocking the growth of cancer cells.

Likewise, foods such as tomatoes, which contain lycopene, can help reduce the risk of skin cancer. Lycopene is a powerful antioxidant that protects our skin from harmful UV radiation, which can cause skin cancer. Additionally, nuts, seeds, and oily fish, such as salmon, are rich in omega-3 fatty acids, which can help reduce inflammation and lower the risk of skin cancer.

Aside from adopting a healthy lifestyle and consuming cancer-fighting foods, it's crucial to protect our skin from harmful UV rays. This can be done by using sunscreen with a high SPF, wearing protective clothing, and avoiding prolonged exposure to the sun, especially during peak hours.

In conclusion, as someone who has experienced the effects of skin cancer first-hand, I cannot stress enough the importance of adopting a healthy lifestyle and consuming foods that can help prevent skin cancer. While it's essential to protect our skin from UV radiation, we should also focus on building our immune system to fight cancer-causing agents. By taking care of our bodies and making healthier choices, we can significantly reduce the risk of skin cancer and lead a happier, healthier life.

Finally, I want to express my deepest gratitude to all those who supported me throughout my journey of fighting skin cancer. Your love, encouragement, and support has been a source of strength and inspiration to me. I hope this cookbook has provided valuable information on how to reduce the risk of skin cancer and encourages you to make healthier choices for yourself and your loved ones. Remember, prevention is always better than cure. Let us all commit to a healthier and happier lifestyle!

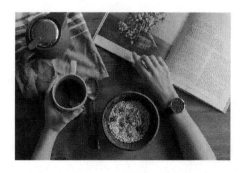

NOTES

Made in the USA
Las Vegas, NV
16 February 2024

85860063R00111